MEDICAL
ABBREVIATIONS
DICTIONARY

MEDICAL ABBREVIATIONS DICTIONARY

(M.A.D)

Dr David Daniel Falijala
WALUUBE

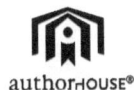

authorHOUSE®

AuthorHouse™
1663 Liberty Drive
Bloomington, IN 47403
www.authorhouse.com
Phone: 1-800-839-8640

First published by AuthorHouse   08/25/2011

ISBN: 978-1-4567-8497-3 (sc)

Printed in the United States of America

Edited by: Dr David Daniel Falijala WALUUBE: M.B.Ch.B; DA; MRCA (U.K).
No 6 Pennine Way, Downswood, Maidstone, Kent, ME 15 8 UG. U.K.
Tel. No + 44(1622) 862744. E-mail dwaluube@hotmail.co.uk

CONTENTS

Dedicated to *Mary my wife; Mary Nalweiso my mother; my children and in memory of my late uncle Dr David Falijala Ibanda.*

PREFACE

This Dictionary of Medical Abbreviations aims at providing up-to-date meaning of abbreviations used in medical literature written by medical and scientific professionals, mainly in the U.K. Most medical abbreviations are speciality-specific and most specialities have their own batch of hieroglyphics. Not all abbreviations listed here are Internationally recognised and used nor recommended.

This dictionary will appeal to medical professionals in Overseas English-speaking countries, who regularly access books and journals from the U.K and the USA; and to those professionals who visit the U.K for various professional meetings and activities. An Abbreviations Dictionary cannot be comprehensive as the written format of medical notation evolves naturally with time and with individual author's "idiosyncrasies". I recommend it to those medical professionals most perplexed by Abbreviations.

References have not been included as these Abbreviations were compiled from multiple sources, including National and International Journals, Textbooks and lectures.

ACKNOWLEDGEMENTS

I wish to thank Ms Sharon Blackmore of Directorate of Anaesthesia and Critical Care at the William Harvey Hospital, Ashford, Kent,U.K, for her efforts to get this book published, and I am grateful to Ms Sarah Oogden, Commissioning Editor at the Royal College of Medicine, for her advice. I thank the Library staff at the William Harvey Hospital Postgraduate Centre, for all the help given to me during my editing of this book.

INTRODUCTION

The dictionary contains abbreviations currently in use in English-speaking countries but emphasis has been on covering those used in the U.K and the USA.

The Dictionary is arranged in alphabetical order and most of the abbreviations start with a capital letter. Some abbreviations are followed by small letters in brackets. The following statement or description for the abbreviation starts with a capital letter even for those abbreviations in smalll letters.

Countries, outside of the U.K, where some of the abbreviations are commonly used, have been identified in brackets and I have used spellings used in each specific country. Some abbreviations may not be used much by relevant medical specialities. Some new abbreviations will come up as a result of medical and scientific advances and due to National and International administrative policy changes. Scientific advances will always set the pace.

a (aa)	: Artery (Arteries).
As	: Adenoids/Adenoidectomy.
A2	: Aortic second heart sound.
A 3	: Beta Amyloid.
AA	: Alcoholics Anonymous.
	Amino Acid.
	Ascending Aorta
	Atomic Absorption.
	Australian Antigen.
A2A	: Angiotensin-2-Antagonist.
AAA	: Abdominal Aortic Aneurysm
	Asleep—Awake—Asleep.
	Aspirin for Asymptomatic Atherosclerosis.
AAAHC	: Accreditation Association for Ambulatory Health Care. (USA).
AAAASF	: American Association for Accreditation of Ambulatory Surgery Facilities.
AABB	: American Association of Blood Banks.
AACI	: Arachidonic Acid Cascade Inhibitor.
AAFB	: Acid-Alcohol-Fast Bacillus.
AAGBI	: Association of Anaesthetists of Great Britain and Ireland.
AAGL	: American Association of Gynecologic Laparoscopists.
AAI	: A-line Retrogressive Index.
AAL	: Anterior Axillary Line.
AAMCs	: Association of American Medical Colleges. (USA).
AAMI	: Age-Associated Memory Impairment.
AAPHelp	: Acute Abdominal Pain Help.(Ref. Structured proforma for checking patients).
AAS	: Admission Avoidance Scheme.
	Anthrax Anti-serum.
AAV	: Adeno-Associated Virus.
Ab	: Antibody.
AB	: Accesory Breast.
	Axio-buccal.
ABC	: Activities-specific Balance Confidence.
	Airway; Breathing and Circulation.
	Aneurysmal Bone Cyst.

ABCD : Airway, Breathing, Circulation, Disability.
Association of British Clinical Diabetologists.
ABCDE : Airway; Breathing; Circulation; Disability Exposure.
ABCIC : Airway, Breathing, Circulation, Intravenous Crystolloid.
ABD : Autologous Blood Donation.
ABE : Actual Base Excess.
ABFG : Aorto-Bifemoral Graft.
ABG(ABGs) : Arterial Blood Gases.
ABH : Actual Bodily Harm.
ABI : Absolute Benefit Increase.
ABP : Acute Blood Purification.
ABPA : Allergic Bronchopulmonary Aspergillosis.
ABPI : Ankle-Brachial Pressure Index. (Ref. ratio between highest systolic Ankle and Brachial Blood Pressure).
Association of the British Pharmaceutical Industry.
ABPN : Association of British Paediatric Association.
ABR : Ankle to Brachial Ratio.
Auditory Brain Stem Evoked Response.
ABRA : American Blood Resources Association.
ABRHP : Advisory Board on the Registration of Homoeopathic Products.
ABRS : Acute Bacterial Rhinosinusitis.
ABS : Amniotic Band Syndrome.
Apical Ballooning Syndrome. (Ref. ischaemic pain without Coronary Artery Disease).
Analgesia-Based Sedation.
AbSD : Abductor-type Spasmodic Dysphonia.
ABV : Alcohol by Volume (percentage of).
ABx : Antibiotics.

AC : Abdominal Circumference.
Acromio-clavicular.
Air Conduction.
Alternating Current.
Approved Clinician.
Audit Commission.
ac (a/c) : Ante cibum. (Ref. Latin for "before food").
ACA : Anterior Cerebral Artery.

	Anti-Centromere Antibody.
	Association for Continence Advice.
ACAD	: Ambulatory Care and Diagnostic (Unit).
ACBS	: Advisory Committee on Borderline Substances.
ACBT	: Active Cycle of Breathing Techniques.
ACC	: Abdominal Aortic Cross-Clamping.
	Adenoid Cyst Carcinoma.
ACCEA	: Advisory Committee on Clinical Excellence Awards.
ACCHN	: Adenoid Cyst Carcinoma of Head and Neck.
anti-CCP	: Anti-cyclic Citrullinated Peptide (antibodies).
ACCS	: Acute Care Common Stem.
	Acute Common Care Stem. (USA).
ACCT	: Assessment Care in Custody and Teamwork.
ACD	: Acid Citrate Dextrose.
	Allergic Contact Dermititis.
	Anaemia of Chronic Disease.
	Anaesthetic Conserving Device.
ACDA	: Advisory Committee on Distinction Awards.
ACDP	: Advisory Committee on Dangerous Pathogens.
ACE	: Advanced Combined Encoder.
	Aerosol Cloud Enhancer.
	Angiotensin Converting Enzyme.
	Antegrade Continent Enema.
	Autologous-Cultured Epithelium.
ACEIs	: Angiotensin Converting Enzyme Inhibitors.
ACEVO	: Association of Chief Executives of Voluntary
	Organisations.
ACF	: Academic Clinical Fellowship.
	Ante-Cubital Fossa.
ACGME	: Accreditation Council on Graduate Medical Education.
ACGT	: Advisory Committee on Generic Testing.
ACh.	: Acetylcholine.
ACH	: Adrenocortical Hormone.
	Ambulatory Care Hospital.
AChEIs	: Acetylcholinesterase Inhibitors.
AChRs	: Acetylcholine Receptors.
ACJ	: Acromioclavicular Joint.
aCL	: Anti-Cardiolipin Antibody.

ACL	: Anterior Cruciate Ligament.
ACLA	: Anti-Cardiolipin Antibodies.
ACLF	: Acute on Chronic Liver Failure.
ACLR	: Anterior Cruciate Ligament Reconstruction.
ACLS	: Advanced Cardiac Life Support.
ACMD	: Advisory Council on Misuse of Drugs.
ACNFP	: Advisory Committee on Novel Foods and Substances.
ACON	: Anaesthetic Areas of Concern/Consideration.
ACOVE	: Assessing Care of Vulnerable Elders.
ACP	: Augmented Care Period.
ACPRC	: Association of Chartered Physiotherapists in Respiratory Care.
ACPS	: Acrocephalopolysyndactyly Syndrome.
ACR	: Albumin: Creatinine Ratio. Anticoagulation Reversal.
ACRA	: Advisory Committee on Resource Allocation.
ACRAb	: Acetylcholine Receptor Antibodies.
ACS	: Abdominal Compartment Syndrome. Acute Compartment Syndrome. Acute Coronary Syndrome. Acute Chest Syndrome.(Ref. pulmonary complication in Sickle Cell Disease).
ACSF	: Artificial Cerebrospinal Fluid.
ACSM	: American College of Sports Medicine.
ACT	: Activated Clotting Time. Additional Contribution to Training (Medical) Assertive Community Treatment.
ACTA	: Association of Cardiothoracic Anaesthetists.
ACTG	: **AIDS** Clinical Trials Group. (USA).
ACTH	: Adrenocorticotrophic Hormone.
ACT-LR	: Activated Clotting Time-Low Range.
ACV	: Assist Control Ventilation.
AD	: Adrenaline. Alzheimer`s Dementia (or Disease). Autogenic Drainage. Autosomal Dominant (inheritance).
ADA	: Adenosine De-Aminase.

	American Diabetes Association.
	American Dietetic Association.
ADAMHA	: Alcohol, Drug Abuse, and Mental Health Administration.
ADAPT	: Association for Drug Abuse Prevention and Treatment.
ADC	: Adult Diabetes Care.
	AIDS Dementia Complex.
	Apparent Diffusion Co-efficient.
ADCC	: Antibody-Dependent Cellular Cytotoxicity.
ADD	: Attention Deficit Disorder.
ADDH	: Attention Deficit Disorder with Hyperactivity.
AdDT	: Adolescent Diabetes Intervention Trial.
ADEM	: Acute Disseminated Encephalomyelitis.
ADFAM	: Aid for Addicts and Family.
ADI	: Acceptable Daily Intake.
	Adverse Drug Interaction.
ad.lib.	: Ad libitum. (Ref. Latin for; "as much/as often as wanted").
ADH	: Anti-diuretic Hormone.
ADHD	: Attention Deficit Hyperactivity Disorder.
ADHR	: Autosomal Dominant Hypophosphataemic Rickets.
ADJ	: Amelo-Dentinal Junction.
ADL	: Activities of Daily Living (or Aids to Daily Living).
ADM	: Adrenomedullin. (Ref. a potent vasodilator Factor).
ADOD	: Arthrodentosteodysplasia.
ADP	: Accidental Dural Puncture.
	Adenosine Diphosphate.
ADPKD	: Autosomal Dominant Polycystic Kidney.
ADROIT	: Adverse Drug Reactions Online Information Tracking.
ADQ	: Augmented-delta-quotient.
ADQI	: Acute Dialysis Quality Initiative.
ADR	: Adverse Drug Reaction.
	Alternative Dispute Resolution.
ADRT	: Advance Decision to Refuse Treatment.
ADSS	: Association of Directors of Social Services.
ADT	: Accepted Dental Therapeutics.
AEs	: Adverse Experiences.
A & E	: Accident and Emergency.

AEA	: Above-the-Elbow Amputation.
AEB	: As Evidenced by.
AEC	: Airway Exchange Catheter.
AECG	: Ambulatory **ECG.**
AEDS(AEDs)	: Anti-Epilepsy Drugs.
	Automated (or Automatic) External Defibrillators.
AEMT	: Association of Emergency Medical Technicians.
AEP	: Auditory Evoked Potential.
AEPs	: Auditory Evoked Potentials. (Ref. used to monitor intra-ocular pressure).
Aet	: Aetas. (Ref. Latin for Age).
AF	: Ameloblastic Fibroma.
	Amniotic Fluid.
	Anal Fissure.
	Apical Foramen.
	Atrial Fibrillation.
AFA	: **AIDS** Follow-up Assessment.
AFAR	: American Federation for Aging Research.
AFB	: Acid-Fast Bacilli.
	Aorto-Femoral Bypass.
AFE	: Amniotic Fluid Embolism.
AFH	: Angiomatoid Fibrous Histiocytoma.
AFI	: Amniotic Fluid Index.
AFFIRM	: Atrial Fibrillation Follow-up Investigation of Rhythm Management.
AFLP	: Acute Fatty Liver of Pregnancy.
AFNs	: Adapting Firing Neurones. (Ref. spinal dorsal neurones).
AFP	: Alpha-Foeto-Protein.
AFPRB	: Armed Forces Pay Review Body.
AFS	: Allergic Fungal Sinusitis.
AFT	: Autologous Fat Transfer.
AFV	: Amniotic Fluid Volume.
Ag	: Antigen.
AG	: Anion Gap. (Ref. in Acid-Base disorders).
A/G	: Albumin: Globulin (Ratio).
AGA	: Androgenic Alopecia.

Appropriate for Gestational Age.

AGC : Aspartate-Glutarnate Carrier.

AGF : Autologous Growth Factor.

AGNB : Anaerobic Gram-negative Bacilli.

AGREE : Appraisal of Guidelines Research and Evaluation.

AGT : Angiotensin.

AGUS : Atypical Glandular Cell of Undetermined Significance.

AHA : Alpha-Hydroxy Acid.
Area Health Authority.

AHCPR : Agency for Health Care Policy and Research. (Now, **AHRQ**).

AHF : Acute Heart Failure.
Anti-Haemophilic Factor.

AHI : Apnoea-hypopnoea Index. (Ref. events of apnoea per hour of sleep).
Arthritis Helplessness Index.

AHO : Albright Hereditary Osteodystrophy.

AHP : Allied Health Professional.

AHR : Airway Hyperesponsiveness (or Airway Hyper-Reactivity).

AHRQ : Agency for Healthcare Research and Quality. (Previously, **AHCPR**).

AHSC : Academic Health Sciences Centre.

AHTR : Acute Haemolytic Transfusion Reaction.

AI : Adequate Intake.
Aortic Insufficiency.
Artificial Insemination.

AIA : **AIDS** Initial Assessment.

AIC : Akaike Information Criterion. (Ref. risk assessment in hip operations).
Aintree Intubation Catheter.(Ref. aid in Fibreoptic Intubation Thru **LMA**).

AICA : Anterior Inferior Cerebellar Artery.

AICD : Automatic Implantable Cardioverter Defibrillator.

AICR : Association for International Cancer Research.

AICU : Adult Intensive Care Unit.

AID : Artificial Insemination by Donor.
AIDP : Acute Inflammatory Demyelinating
Polyradiculoneuropathy.
AIDS : Acquired Immuno-Deficiency Syndrome.
AIED : Autoimmune Inner Ear Disease.
AIH : Artificial Insemination by Husband.
Auto-Immune Hepatitis.
AIHA : Auto-Immune Haemolytic Anaemia.
AIM : Inadequate Responders to Methotrexate.
Anaesthesia in Management.
AIMS : Abnormal Involuntary Movement Scale.
Association for Improvements in the Maternity Services.
AIMSW : Associate of the Institute of Medical Social Workers.
AIN : Acute Interstitial Nephritis.
Anal Intraepithelial Neoplasia.
Auto-Immune Neutropenia.
AIP : Acute Interstitial Pneumonia.
AIPHTN : Acute Intra-operative Pulmonary Hypertension.
AIRE : Autoimmune Regulator Gene.
AIS : Abbreviated Injury Scale.
Adenocarcinoma in situ.
AITFL : Anterior-Inferior Tibial Fibular Ligament.
AITP : Autoimmune Thrombocytopenia Purpura.

AJCC : American Joint Committee on Cancer.
AJDO : Arterio-Jugular Oxygen Content Difference.
AJP : American Journal of Psychiatry.
AJN : American Journal of Nursing.

AK : Actinic Keratoses.
AKA : Above-the-Knee Amputation.
Alcoholic Keto-acidosis.
Also Known As.
AKI : Acute Kidney Injury.
AKIN : Acute Kidney Injury Network (Guidelines).

Al : Aluminium.
AL : Axial Length.

ALA	: Aminolevulinic Acid.
ALACT	: Action;Looking back;Awareness; Creating; Trial. (Ref. a Teaching method).
ALARP	: As Low As Reasonably Possible/Practicable. (Ref. Radiology exposures).
Alb	: Albumin.
ALD	: Alcoholic Liver Disease. Adrenoleucodystrophy.
ALDH	: Aldehyde Dehydrogenase.
ALF	: Acute Liver Failure.
ALI	: Acute Lung Injury.
ALL	: Acute Lymphoblastic Leukaemia.
ALLHAT	: Anti-hypertensive and Lipid-lowering treatment to prevent Heart Attack Trial.
ALM	: Acral Lentiginous Melanoma.
ALOs	: Actinomycosis-like Organisms.
ALP	: Alkaline Phosphatase.
ALRI	: Acute Lower Respiratory Infection.
ALS	: Advanced Life Support. Amyotrophic Lateral Sclerosis.
ALSO	: Advanced Life Support Obstretics.
ALT	: Alanine Aminotransferase.
ALTENS	: Acupuncture-like Transcutaneous Electric Nerve Stimulation.
AMA	: Against Medical Advice. American Medical Association.(USA). Anti-Mitochondrial Antibodies.
AMABO	: Association of Medical Advisers to British Orchestras.
AMAN	: Acute Motor Axonal Neuropathy.
Amb	: Ambulance.
AMC	: Academic Medical Center. (USA). Arthrogryposis Multiplex Congenita.
AMCP	: Academy of Managed Care Pharmacy. (USA)
AMD	: Age-related Macular Degeneration (or Disease). Airway Management Device.
AME	: Airway Medical Equipment.
AMETOP	: Amethocaine Topical Local Anaesthetic.

AMG	: Acceleromyography. (Ref. a test for residual neuro-muscular blockade).
AMH	: Anti-Mullerian Hormone.
AMHP	: Approved Mental Health Professionals.
AMI	: Acute Myocardial Infarction.
	Acute Myocardial Ischaemia.
	Anterior Myocardial Infarction.
AML	: Acute Myeloblastic Leukaemia.
	Acute Myelocytic Leukaemia.
	Acute Myelogenous Leukaemia.
	Acute Myeloid Leukaemia.
	Anterior Midsternal Line.
	Anterior Mitral Leaflet.
AMN	: Adrenomyloneuropathy.
AMOH	: Association of Medical Officers of Health.
amp	: Amputation.
AMP	: Adenosine Monophosphate.
AMPA	: Alpha-amino 3-hydroxy-5-methyl-4-Isoxazole Propionic Acid.
AMPLE	: Allergies, Medications, Past medical history, Last meal,Events leading to presentation.
AMPT	: Alpha-methyl-p-Tyrosine.
AMS	: Acute Mountain Sickness.
	Ablepharon Macrostomia.
	Altered Mental Status.
AMSAN	: Acute Motor and Sensory Axonal Neuropathy.
AMTS	: Abridged Mental Test Score.
	Abbreviated Mental Test Score.
AMU	: Acute Medical Unit.
AN	: Acoustic Neuroma.
	Anorexia Nervosa.
	Antenatal.
	Avascular Necrosis.(see under **AVN**).
ANA	: American Nurses Association.
	Anti-nuclear Antibodies. (Ref. in **SLE** testing).
ANAE	: Alpha-Naphthyl Acetate Esterase.

ANARP	: Alcohol Needs Assessment Research Project. (Ref. General Practice Research).
Anat.	: Anatomy.
ANC	: Absolute Neutrophil Count. Antenatal Clinic.
ANCA	: Anti-Neutrophilic-Cytoplasmic Antibody.
ANCAs	: Anti-Neutrophil Cytoplasmic Antibody-Associated (Disorders). Anti-Nuclear Cytoplasmatic Antibodies. (Ref. **IgG** Antibodies seen in Pregnancy and in Wegener`s Granulomatosis Disease).
ANCOVA	: Analysis of Covariance. (USA).
ANCPIC	: Australian`s National Cannabis Prevention and Information Centre.
AND	: Allow Natural Death.
ANDAs	: Abbreviated Drug Applications.
ANDI	: Abnormalities (or Aberrations) of Normal Development and Involution.
ANF	: Anti-Nuclear Factor.
ANH	: Acute Normovolaemic Haemorrhage. Artificial Nutrition and Hydration.
ANLL	: Acute Non-lymphoblastic Leukaemia.
ANN	: Artificial Neuro-Network. (Ref. for predicting **PONV**).
ANNP	: Advanced Neonatal Nurse Practitioner.
ANOVA	: Analysis of Variance. (Ref. a Statistics model).
ANP	: Atrial Natriuretic Peptides.(Ref. cardiac myocytes in vascular endothelium).
ANPs	: Advanced Nurse Practitioners.
ANS	: Anterior Nasal Spine (of the Hard Palate). Autonomic Nervous System.
ANSA	: Association for Nurses in Substance Abuse.
ant.	: Anterior.
ANTS	: Anaesthesia Non-Technical Skills.(Ref. safety system in **ICU** and Theatres). Acute Neonatal Transport Service.
ANUG	: Acute Necrotising Ulcerative Gingivitis.
Ao	: Aorta.

AoDP	: Aortic Diastolic Pressure.
AOM	: Acute Otitis Media.
AOMRC	: Academy of Medical Royal Colleges.
AOT	: Adenomatoid Odontogenic Tumour.
AP	: Amyloid Plaques.
	Anaesthesia Practitioner.
	Antero-Posterior.
	Apical Pulse.
	Assault Precautions
APs	: Anti-Platelets.
APA	: Association of Paediatric Anaesthetists.
	American Psychiatric Association.
APACHE	: Acute Physiology And Chronic Health Evaluation.
APAIS	: Amsterdam Pre-operative Anxiety and Information Scale.
APB	: Abductor Pollicis Brevis.
aPC	: Activated Protein C.
APC	: Adenomatosis Polyposis Coli (gene).
	Anaesthetic-induced Preconditioning.(Ref. in Gas-induced Anaesthesia).
	Antigen-presenting Cell.
APCR	: Activated Protein C Resistance.
APD	: Adult Polycystic Disease.
	Afferent Pupillary Defect.
	Ambulatory Peritoneal Dialysis.
	Antisocial Personality Disorder.
	Auditory Processing Disorder.
	Automated Peritoneal Dialysis.
APDs	: Anti-Platelet Drugs.
APE	: Approximate Entropy.
APECED	: Autoimmune Polyendocrinopathy-Candidiasis-Ectodermal Dystrophy.
APER	: Abdomino-Perineal Excision of the Rectum.
APGAR	: American Paediatric Gross Assessment Record (Score). (Ref. Appearance, Pulse, Grimace (or Reflexes), Activity, Respiratory effort).
APH	: Ante-Partum Haemorrhage.
APIE	: Assessment, Plan, Intervention, Evaluation.

APKD	: Adult Polycystic Kidney Disease.
APKG	: Acute Primary Keratotic Gingivostomatitis.
APL	: Abductor Pollicis Longus.
	Antiphospholipid.
	Automated Pressure Limiting.
APLA	: Anti-Phospholipid Antibody.
APLS	: Advanced Paediatric Life Support.
APLV	: Adjustable Pressure Limiting Valve.(Ref. used in Anaesthetic equipments).
APML	: Acute Polymyelocystic Leukaemia.
APMS	: Alternative Provider Medical Services.
APN	: Artificial Pneumothorax.
Apo	: Apolipoprotein
APOE(ApoE)	: Apolipoprotein E.(Ref. a major genetic locus for Alzheimer`s Disease).
APP	: Amyloid Precursor Protein.
APPG	: All-Party Pharmacy Group.
Approx.	: Approximately.
APRV	: Airway Pressure Release Ventilation.
APS	: Acute Pain Services.
	Anti-phospholipid (Antibody) Syndrome.
	Autoimmune Polyendocrine Syndromes.(Ref. Type 1 **APECED** and Type 11 **Schmidtt`s** Syndromes).
APSAC	: Anisoylated Plasminogen-Streptokinase Activator Complex (or Anistreplase).
APTC	: Anti-Platelet Trialists Collaboration.(Ref. to the criteria for medical adverse experiences).
APTR	: Activated Prothrombin Partial Thromboplastin Ratio.
APTT	: Activated Partial Thromboplastin Time.
APTTR (APTTr)	: Activated Partial Thromboplastin Time Ratio.
APUD (APUDomas.)	: Amine Precursor Uptake and Decarboxylase (Cells).
AQP4	: Anti-aquaporin 4 (antibodies.):(Ref. in Acute myelopathy in pregnancy and in Neuromylitis Optica.)
AR	: Acoustic Rhinometry.
	Aortic Regurgitation.

Attributable Risk.
Autosomal Recessive (inheritance).
A-R : Apical-Radial (Pulse).
ARA : Angiotensin-Receptor Antagonist.
American Rheumatology Association.
Automated Remifentanil Alogarithm (system).
ARBs (A2RBs): Angiotensin 11 Receptor Blockers.
ARC : **AIDS**-related Complex.
Arthritis Reasearch Campaign.
Arthritis and Rheumatism Council.
ARCL : Accepted Red Blood Cell Loss.
ARCP : Annual Review of Competence.
ARDD : Alcohol-Related Developmental Disability.
ARDS : Acute Respiratory Distress Syndrome.
Adult Respiratory Distress Syndrome.
ARF : Acute Renal Failure.
Acute Respiratory Failure.
Annual Retention Fee (of the **GMC**).
Attributable Risk Fraction.
ARI : Absolute Risk Increase.
Acute Respiratory Infection.
ARM : Artificial Rupture of Membranes.
ARMA : Arthritis and Musculoskeletal Alliance.
ARND : Alcohol-Related Neurodevelopmental Disorder.
AROM : Active Range of Motion.
Artificial Rupture of the Membranes.
ARP : Atrial Refractory Period.
ARR : Absolute Risk Reduction..
ARRP : AnatomicRetropubic Prostatectomy.
ARS : Anaesthetic Research Society.
ARSAC : Administration of Radioactive Substances Advisory
Committee. (USA).
ART : Accredited Record Technician.
Anti-Retroviral Treatment.
Antiviral Therapy.
Assisted Reproduction Technology (or Techniques).
ARVs : Anti-Retrovirals; (Drugs).
ARVD : Atherosclerotic Renovascular Disease.

ARVD/C	: Arrhythmogenic Right Ventricular Dysplasia/ Cardiomyopathy.
AS	: AlimentarySystem.
	Ankylosing Spondylitis.
	Aortic Stenosis.
5-ASA	: 5-Aminosalicyclic Acid.
ASA	: Acetyl salcylic Acid.
	Adaptive Speech Alignment.
	Advertising Standards Agency.
	American Society of Anesthesiologists.
ASAP	: As Soon As Possible
ASCC	: Additional Supply Capability and Capacity.
ASCO	: American Society of Clinical Oncology.
ASCVD	: Arteriosclerotic Heart Disease.
ASD	: Acute Stress Disorder.
	Atrial Septal Defect.
	Autism Spectrum Disorders.
ASDH	: Acute Sub-dural Haematoma.
ASES	: Arthritis Self-Efficacy Scale.
ASSET	: Athena Survey of Science, Engineering and Technology.
ASH	: Action on Smoking and Health.
	Asymmetrical Septal Hypertrophy.
ASI	: Anxiety Status Inventory.
ASIF	: Association for the Study of Internal Fixation.
ASIS	: Anterior Superior Iliac Spine.
ASMA	: Anti-Smooth Muscle Antibody.
ASSIST	: Assessment Score for Sick-patient Identification and Set-up in Treatment.
ASO	: Antistreptolysis-O (Titre.)
	Arteriosclerosis Obliterans.
ASOT	: Anti-Streptolysin-O-Titre.
ASPAN	: American Society of Post-Anesthesia Nurses.
ASPS	: Alveolar Soft Part Sarcoma.
ASSI	: Accurate Surgical and Scientific Instruments.
AST	: Alcohol Sniff Test.
	Aspartate Amino-Transaminase.
ASTMS	: Association of Scientific Technical and Managerial Staffs.

ASU	: Ambulatory Surgery Unit.
asx	: Asymptomatic.
ASW	: Approved Social Worker.
AT	: AnaerobicThreshold.(Ref. in pre-operative assessment for major surgery).
	Anti-Thrombin.
	Assistive Technology.
	Atrial Tachycardia.
AT 11	: Angiotensin 11
ATC	: Anaplastic Thyroid Carcinoma.
ATF	: Alcohol, Tobacco, and Firearms.
ATFL	: Anterior Talofibular Ligament.
ATG	: Antithymocyte Globulin. (Ref. in the induction of lymphopenia).
ATLS	: Acute Tumour Lysis Syndrome.
	Advanced Trauma Life Support.
ATM	: Abbreviated Mental Test.
ATN	: Acute Tubular Necrosis.
ATP	: Adenosine Triphosphate.
	Alloimmune Thrombocytopenic Purpura.
	Ambient Temperature and Pressure.
ATPS	: Ambient Temperature and Pressure Saturated.
ATRA	: All-Trans-Retinoic Acid.
ATS	: Anti-Tetanus Serum.
ATT	: Anti-Thrombotic Trialists Collaboration.
ATTC	: Anti-Thrombotic Treatment Trialists Collaboration.
AUC	: Area Under the Curve. (Ref. in Statistics).
AUDIT	: Alcohol Use Disorders Identification Test.
AUG	: Acute Ulcerative Gingivitis.
AUGIS	: Association of Upper Gastrointestinal Surgeons.
AUR	: Acute Urinary Retention.
Ausc	: Auscultation.
Aux	: Auxiliary.
A-V	: Arterio-Venous.
	Atrio-Ventricular (Node or Bundle).

AVA	: Aortic Valve Area.
	Arterio-Venous Anastomosis.
AVB	: Atrio-Ventricular Block.
AVERT	: Aids Education and Research Trust.
aVF	: Augmented Voltage Lead Left Leg.
AVF	: Arterio-Venous Fistula.
AVGC	: Autogenous Vein Graft Conduit.
aVL	: Augmented Voltage Lead Left Arm.
AVM	: Arterio-Venous Malformation.
	Atrio-Ventricular Malformation.
AVN	: Atrial Ventricular Node.
	Avascular Necrosis.
AVNRT	: Atrio-Ventricular Nodal Re-entry Tachycardia.
	Atrio-Ventricular Nodal Reciprocating Tachycardia.
AVO	: Aortic Valve Opening.
a-vO₂ diff.	: Arterio-Venous oxygen concentration difference.
AVP	: Arginine Vasopressin.
AVPU	: Alert;Verbal;Pain-responsive;Unresponsive.(Ref. Consciousness level Test).
aVR	: Augmented Voltage Right Arm.
AVR	: Aortic Valve Replacement.
AVRT	: Atrio-Ventricular Reentrant Tachycardia.
AVSD	: Atrioventricular Renovascular Disease.
AVVs	: Atrial Ventricular Valves.
AW	: Awake. (Ref. recovery from General Anaesthesia).
A & W	: Alive and Well.
AWB	: Autologous Whole Blood.
AWS	: Airway Scope. (Ref. Anaesthetic Fibreoptic Intubating Device).
Ax	: Aortic Cross-Clamping.
AXR	: Abdominal X-Ray.
AXR(e & s)	: Abdominal X-Ray (erect & supine).
AZA	: Azathioprine.
AZT	: Azithromycin.
	Azidothymidine. (Generic name is Zidovudine).

B12	: Vitamin B12.
Ba	: Barium.
BAAPS	: British Association of Aesthetic Plastic Surgeons.
BAC	: Blood Alcohol Concentration.
BACUP	: British Association of Cancer United Patients.
BAD	: British Association of Dermatologists.
BADGER	: Birmingham and District General Practice Emergency Rooms.
BADS	: British Association of Day Surgery.
BaE	: Barium Enema.
BAEP	: Brain Stem Auditory Evoked Potential.
BAHA	: Bone-anchored Hearing Aid.
BAL	: Balanced Anaesthesia.
BALF	: Brocho-alveolar Lavage Fluid.
BALP	: Bone-specific Alkaline Phosphate.
BAMM	: British Association of Medical Managers.
BAMPS	: Bilateral Auterolateral Magnetic Stimulation (Technique).
BAN	: British Approved Name.
BAOMS	: British Association of Oral and Maxillofacial Surgeons.
BAON	: British Association of Orthopaedic Nurses.
BAPAM	: British Association for Performing Art Medicine.
BAPEN	: British Association for Parenteral and Enteral Nutrition.
BAPS	: Biomechanical Ankle Platform System.
BAPW	: British Association of Pharmaceutical Wholesalers.
BARS	: Barnes Akathisia Rating Scale.(Ref. tool for detection and monitoring of Akathisia in patients on **TCAs**; **MAOIs; SSRIs; 5-HTs** psychiatric drugs).
BAS 11	: British Ability Scales 11.
BASIC	: British Association for Immediate Care.
BASICS	: British Association for Immediate Care Scotland.
BASDAI	: Bath Ankylosing Spondylitis Disease Activity Index.
BASFI	: Bath Ankylosing Spondylitis Function Index.
BAS-G	: Bath Ankylosing Spondylitis Global.
BASMI	: Bath Ankylosing Spondylitis Measurement Index.
BASP	: British Association of Stroke Physicians.
BAT	: Basophil Activation Test. Brown Adipose Tissue.

BAUP	: Bovie-assisted Uvulopalatoplasty.
BAV	: Bicuspid Aortic Valve. (Ref. a congenital cardiac anomaly).
BAVQ	: Beliefs About Voices Questionnaire.
BAWO	: Bilateral Antral Washouts.
BB	: Bronchial Blockers.
BBA	: Born Before Arrival.
BBB	: Blood Brain Barrier. Bundle Branch Block.
BBD	: Baby Born Dead.
BBP	: Blood-borne Pathogens.
BBSRC	: Biotechnology and Biological Sciences Research Council.
BBV	: Blood-borne Virus.
BC	: Blood Culture. Bone Conduction. Breathing Control.
BCA	: British Chiropractic Association.
BCAA	: Branched Chain Amino Acids.
BCAO	: Bilateral Carotid Artery Occlusion.
BCC	: Basal Cell Carcinoma.
BCE	: Basal Cell Epithelium.
BCG	: Bacille Calmette-Guerin (vaccine).
BCHA	: Bone Conducting Hearing Aid.
BCIS	: Bone Cement Implantation Syndrome. British Cardiac Intervention Society.
BCLP	: Bilateral Cleft Lip and Palate.
BCLS	: Basic Cardiac Life Support.
BCMA	: Breast Care and Mastectomy Association.
BCOP	: Blood Colloid Osmotic Pressure.
BCP	: Basic Calcium Phosphate. Birth Control Pill.
BCR	: Breakpoint Cluster Region.(Ref. Chromosome 22 in Chronic Myeloid Leukaemia: **CML**).
BCRs	: B-Cell Receptors.
BCS	: British Cardiac Society.
BCSR	: Bone-Conducting Surface Ratio.

BCVA	: Best Corrected Visual Acuity.
bd	: Bis die. (Ref. Latin for "twice daily").
BD	: Bis Die (Ref. Latin for "twice daily"; see **b.d.**).
	Brain Dysfunction.
BDA	: British Dental Association.
	British Diabetic Association.
	British Dietetic Association.
BDDE	: Body Dysmorphic Disorder Examination.
BDI	: Beck`s Depression Inventory.
BDJ	: British Dental Journal.
BDP	: Beclomethasone Diphosphate.
	Brief Dynamic Psychotherapy.
BDS	: Bachelor in Dental Surgery.
BDZ	: Benzodiazepine.
BE	: Barium Enema.
	Base Excess.(see under **BXS**).
BEA	: Below-the-Elbow Amputation.
	British Epilepsy Association.
BEAR	: Brain Stem Evoked Auditory Response.
BED	: Binge Eating Disorder.
BES	: Bilateral Electrical Stimulation.
BF	: Blood Film.
	Breast-Fed.
BFCS	: Basal Forebrain Cholinergic System.
BFI	: Baby Friendly Initiative.
BFM	: Body Fat Mass.
BHA	: Butylated Hydroxyanisole.
BHAT	: Beta-Blocker Heart Attack Trial.
*B*HCG	: Beta-Human Chorionic Gonadotrophin.
BHF	: Better Hospital Food.
	British Heart Foundation.
BHL	: Bilateral Hilar Lymphadenopathy.
BHMA	: British Holistic Medical Association.
BHP	: Blood Hydrostatic Pressure.
BHR	: Bronchial Hyper-Responsiveness.

BHS	: British Hypertension Society.
BHT	: Butylated Hydroxytoluene.
BI	: Bone Injury.
BIA	: Bioelectrical Analysis.
BIBRA	: British Industrial Biological Research Association.
BiC	: Bicarbonate.
BIC	: Bayes Information Criterion.(Ref. risk index in Hip osteoporotic fractures).
BID	: Brought in Dead.
BIDS	: Bedtime Insulin and Daytime Sulfonylureas.
BIH	: Benign Intracranial Hypertension. Bilateral Inguinal Hernias.
BINA	: Bilateral Intranasal Antrostomy.
BINOCAR	: British Isles Network of Congenital Anomaly Registers.
BINP	: Bilateral Intranasal Polypectomy.
Biochem.	: Biochemistry.
Biol.	: Biology.
BIONJ	: Bisphosphonate-induced Osteo-necrosis of the Jaw.
BIPAP (BiPAP):	Biphasic Positive Airway Pressure.
BIPP	: Bismuth Iodine Paraffin Paste.
BIS	: Bispectral Index (monitor). (Ref. used in monitoring depth of Anaesthesia).
BITA	: British Intravenous Therapy Association.
BITE	: Bulimic Investigatory Test Edinburgh.
BJGP	: British Journal of General Practitioners.
BJ protein	: Bence Jones protein.
BJP	: British Journal of Psychiatry.
BKA	: Below Knee Amputation.
BL	: Broad Ligament. Bucco-lingual.
BLa	: Blood Lactate.
BLL	: Blood Lead Level.
BLS	: Basic Life Support.
BLT	: Bilateral(double) Lung Transplantation.

BM	: Bacterial Meningitis.
	Body Mass.
	Boehringer Mannheim (meter). (Ref. for Capillary blood glucose testing).
	Bone Marrow.
	Bowel Movement.
BMA	: Basaloid Monomorphic Adenoma.
	British Medical Association.
BMD	: Becker Muscular Dystrophy.
	Bone Mineral Density.
BME	: Black and Minority Ethnic (Doctors).
BMEPs	: Black and Minority Ethnic Patients.
BMFs	: Breast Milk Fortifiers.
BMI	: Body Mass Index.
BMJ	: British Medical Journal.
BMP	: Basic Metabolic Panel.
BMPR2	: Bone Morphogenetic Receptor 2.
BMR	: Basal Metabolic Rate.
BMstix	: Blood Monitoring (for Blood Sugar.)
BMS	: Bare Metal Stent. (Ref. Coronary Artery Stents).
	Burning Mouth Syndrome.
BMT	: Bone Marrow Transplant (or Transplantation).
BMZ	: Basic Membrane Zone.
BN	: Bachelor of Nursing.
BNA	: Borderline Nuclear Abnomalities.
BNF	: British Medical Formulary.
BNI	: British Nursing Index.
BNO	: Bowels Not Opened.
BNOE	: Benign Necrotising Otitis Externa.
BNP	: Brain Natriuretic Peptide.
	B-type Nutriuretic Peptide; (a Ventricular dysfunction hormonal marker).
BO	: Bowel Obstruction.
BOA	: Born out of Asepsis.
	British Orthopaedic Association.

BOC	: British Oxygen Company.
BOLD	: Blood Oxygen Level Dependent.
BOO	: Bladder Outflow Obstruction.
	Buccinator Orbicularis Oris.
BOOP	: Bronchiolitis Obliterans Organising Pneumonia.
BOP	: Bilateral Ocipitoparietal (Flap).
BOR	: Bowels Open Regularly.
	Brachial-oto-Renal.
BOS	: Base of Skull.
	Base of Support. (Ref. in Orthopaedics).
BP	: Bedpan.
	Blood Pressure.
	British Pharmacopoeia.
	Bullous Pemphigoid.
BP units	: British Pharmacopoeia units.
BPA	: British Paediatric Association.
BPAD	: Bipolar Affective Disorder.
BPC	: British Pharmaceutical Codex.
BPD	: Bi-Parietal Diameter (of Foetus).
	Bipolar Disorder.
	Borderline Personality Disorder.
	Broncho-Pulmonary Dysplasia.
BPEG	: British Pacing and Electrophysiology Group.
BPF	: Broncho-Pleural Fistula.
BPG	: (2,3) Bisphosphoglycerate.
BPH	: Benign Prostatic Hyperplasia (or Hypertrophy).
BPM (bpm)	: Beats per Minute.
BPOG	: British Psychosocial Oncology Group.
BPPV	: Benign Paroxysmal Positional Vertigo.
BPQ	: Breathing Problems Questionnaire.
BPRS	: Brief Psychiatric Rating Scale.
BPS	: British Pain Society.
BPV	: Benign Positional Vertigo.
Br	: Bronchitis.
BRC	: Biomedical Research Centre.
BRCA	: Breast Cancer Susceptibility genes.

BRD	: Baroreflex Dysfunction.
BRIF	: Bonfils Retromolar Intubation Fibroscope.
BRIOTT	: British Randomised Injectable Opiate Treatment Trial.
BRM	: Biological Response Modifiers.
BRS	: Baro-reflex Sensitivity.
	Behaviour Rating Scale.
BRCS	: British Red Cross Society.
BRUM	: Birmingham Rehabilitation Uptake Maximisation (Study).
BS	: Blood Sugar.
	Bowel Sounds.
	Breath Sounds.
BSA	: Body Surface Area.
	Bovine Serum Albumin.
	Breast Self Awareness.
BSACI	: British Society for Allergy and Clinical Immunology.
BSc	: Bachelor of Science.
BSc(Nurs)	: Butchelor of Science(Nursing).
BSC	: Basal Squamous Carcinoma.
	Bedside Commode.
	Burn Scar Contracture.
BSCCP	: British Society for Colposcopy and Cervical Pathology.
BSCPB	: Bilateral Superficial Cervical Plexus Block.
BSE	: Bovine Spongiform Encephalopathy.
	Breast Self-Examination.
BSER	: Brainstem Evoked Response. (Ref. a hearing test).
BSO	: Bilateral Salpingo-oophrectomy.
B`sp	: Bronchospasm.
BSR	: Burst Suppression Ratio. (Ref. in **ECG** monitoring).
BSS	: Balanced Salt Solution.
	Bernad-Soulier Syndrome.
	Black Silk Suture.
BSSA	: British Sjogren`s Syndrome Association.
BST	: Basic Surgical Training.
BT	: Bleeding Time.
BTA	: British Thyroid Association.

BTB	: Break Through Pain.
BTLS	: Basic Trauma Life Support (Course).
BTPS	: Body Temperature and Pressure Saturated.
BTS	: Blood Transfusion Service.
	British Thoracic Society.
BUD	: Budesonide.
BUN	: Blood Urea Nitrogen.
BURP	: Backwards-Upwards, Rightwards Pressure (on the Thyroid Cartilage).
	(Ref. an Intubating manoeuvre in General Anaesthesia).
BV	: Bacterial Vaginosis.
	Blood Volume.
BVAS	: Birmingham Vasculitis Activity Score.
BVPT	: British Vocabulary Picture Test.
Bx	: Biopsy.
BXO	: Balanitis Xerotica Obliterans.
BXS	: Base Excess. (See under **BE**).
BWS	: Beckwith-Wiedemann Syndrome.
BWt	: Birth Weight.
C	: Celsius; Centigrade.
	Cervical.
Ca++	: Calcium
Ca	: Cancer (or Carcinoma).
CA	: Cancer Antigen.
	Chronological Age
	Carbonic Anhydrase..
	Clinical Apprenticeship.
	Cyclic **AMP.**
C&A	: Child and Adolescent.
CA 125	: Carcinoma Antigen 125.
cABC	: Catastrophic bleeding, Airway, Breathing, Circulation.
CABG	: Coronary Artery Bypass Graft.
CACI	: Computer-Assisted Continuous Infusion.
CACT	: Carnitine-Acylcarnitine Translocase.

CAD	: Chronic Coronary Artery Disease.
	Computer Aided Design.
	Coronary Artery Disease.
CADSIL	: Cerebral Autosomal Dominant Arteriopathy with Subcortical Infarctions.
CAF	: Common Assessment Framework.
	Cytoxan, Adriamycin, Fluorouracil
CAGE	: Cerebral Arterial Gas Embolism.
	Cut down, Annoyed, Guilty Eye-Opener. (Ref. a questionnaire).
CAH	: Chronic Active Hepatitis.
	Congenital Adrenal Hyperplasia.
CAIDE	: Cardiovascular risk factors; Aging and Dementia.
CAL	: Chronic Airflow Limitation.
CAM	: Complementary and Alternative Medicine.
	Confusion Assessment Method.
CAMHS	: Child and Adolescent Mental Health Services.
CAMI	: Carer`s Assessment of Managing Index.
cAMP	: Cyclic Amino-Monophosphate.
CAMS	: Candidate Application Matching System.
CAN	: Camberwell Assessment of Need.
	Cardiac Autonomic Neuropathy.
CANDAs	: Computer Assisted New Drug Applications.
CANS	: Central Auditory Nervous System.
CaO$_2$	: Arterial Oxygen Content.
Cap	: Capsule.
CAP	: College of American Pathologists.
	Community Acquired Pneumonia.
	Chronic Adult Periodonitis.
Ca: P	: Calcium: Phosphate Ratio.
CAPOD	: Community **AIDS** Prevention Outreach Demonstration.
CAPD	: Central Auditory Processing Disorder.
	Continuous Ambulatory Peritoneal Dialysis.
CAPTIM	: Comparison of Angioplasty and Pre-hospital Thrombolysis in Myocardial Infarction.
CAR	: Compensatory Anti-inflammatory Response.
	Constitutive Androstane Receptor.(Ref. a receptor for Uridine-Glucuronyl Transferase: **UGT**).

CARDI	: Coronary Artery Risk Developments in young Adults.
CARE	: Cholesterol and Recurrent Events (Trial).
	Cardiac Anaesthesia Risk Evaluation.
CARP	: Coronary Artery Revascularisation Prophylaxis (Study).
CARS	: Compensatory Anti-inflammatory Response System.
CART	: Classification And Regression Tree (Analysis).
	Cocaine and Amphetamines Regulated Transcript.
CAS	: Children Aid Society. (Ref. a Carrera Programme.)
	Cyclic Anti-depressants.
CAST	: Cardiac Arrythmia Suppression Trial.(Ref. Ventricular premature complex).
CAT	: Coblation-Assisted Tonsillectomy.
	Cognitive Analytical Therapy.
	Combined Approach Tympanoplasty.
	Computerised Adaptive Testing.
	Computer Assisted Tomography.
	Computerised (Computed) Axial Tomography.
	Critical Appraisal Trial.
CATCH	: Cambridgeshire Association to Commission Health.
CATT	: Card Agglutination Trypanosomiasis Test.
CATS	: Clinical Assessment and Treatment Services.
CAVH	: Continuous Arterio-Venous Haemofiltration.
CBAVD	: Congenital Bilateral Absence of the vas deferens.
CBC	: Complete Blood Count.
CBCT	: Cone Beam Computed Tomography.
CBD	: Case-based Discussion.
	Common Bile Duct.
CBER	: Center for Biologics Evaluation and Research. (USA).
CBETS	: Competency-Based Education and Training System. (USA).
CBF	: Cerebral Blood Flow.
CBP	: Chronic Bacterial Prostatitis.
CBR	: Community-based Rehabilitation.
CBSC	: Cord Blood Stem Cells.
CBT	: Cognitive Behavioural Therapy.
CBV	: Cerebral Blood Volume.
CBZ	: Carbimazole.

CC	: Chest Clinic.
	Chief Complaint.
	Collagenuous Colitis.
	Costal Cartilage.
	Creatinine Clearance.
	Critical Care.
CCa++	: Corrected Calcium.
CCAM	: Congenital Cystic Adenomatoid Malformation.
CCB	: Calcium Channel Blocker.
CCBST	: Certificate of Completion of Basic Surgical Training.
CCBT	: Computerised Cognitive Behavioural Therapy.
CCD	: Central Core Disease.
	Charge-Coupled Device.(Ref. a Solid State Sensor used in Radiology).
CCDC	: Consultant in Communicable Disease Control.
CCE	: Capacitative Calcium Entry.
CCF	: Congestive Cardiac Failure.(Chronic Cardiac Failure).
CCG	: Costochondral Graft.
CCH	: Circumscribed Choroidal Haemangioma.
CCHD	: Complex Congenital Heart Disease.
CCHF	: Crimean-Congo Haemorrhagic Fever.
CCI	: Chronically Critically Ill.
	Chronic Constriction Injury.
CCIE	: Counter Current Immuno Electrophoresis.
CCIT	: Consultant Contract Implementation Team.
CCK	: Cholecystokinin.
CCM	: Chronic Care Modes.
CCMS	: Cerebrocostomandibular Syndrome.
CCOT	: Clear Cell Odontogenic Tumour.
CCP	: Centre for Clinical Practice.
	Clinical Care Pathway.
	Co-operation and Competition Panel.
CCPD	: Continuous Cyclic Peritoneal Dialysis.
CCR	: Canadian Cervical-Spine Rule.
CCS	: Community Clinical Sciences (Division.)
CCSC	: Central Consultants Specialist Committee.
CCSF	: Carotid-Cavernous Sinus Fistula.

CCST	: Certificate of Completion of Specialist Training.
CCT	: Certificate of Completion of Training.
	Controlled Clinical Trial.
	Controlled Cord Traction. (Ref. in Obstetrics).
	Craniopagus Conjoint Twins.
	Corrected Colour Temperature.(Ref. measured by light from **LEDs**).
CCU	: Cancer Cell Unit.
	Cardiac Care Unit (or Coronary Care Unit).
CCVR	: Combined Contraceptive Vaginal Ring.
CD	: Chemical Dependence.
	Clostridium difficile.
	Cluster of Differentiation.
	Conduct Disorder.
	Controlled Drug.
	Crohn`s Disease.
CD4	: Cluster of Differentiation 4. (see under **CD4T**).
CDs	: Controlled Drugs.
CDA	: Clinical Document Architecture.
CDAD	: Clostridium deficile-Associated Disease (or Diarrhoea).
CDAI	: Crohn`s Disease Activity Index.
CDC	: Centers for Disease Control. (USA).
	Clinical Data Coordinator. (USA).
	Communicable Disease Centres.
	Communicable Disease Control.
CDCP	: Centres for Disease Control and Prevention.
CDGP	: Constitutional Delay in Growth and Puberty.
CDH	: Congenital Dislocation of the Hip.
	Congenital Diaphragmatic Hernia.
CDI	: Central Diabetes Inspidus.
CDO	: Chief Dental Officer.
CDP	: Child Development Programme.
	Clinical Development Plan.
	Continuous Distending Pressure.
	Computerised Dynamic Posturography.
CDR	: Controlled Drug Register.
CDS	: Clinical Decision Support.
	Community Dental Service.

CDSC   : Communicable Disease Survillance Centre.
CDSM   : Committee on Dental and Surgical Materials.
CDSR   : Cochrane Database of Systematic Reviews.
CDSS   : Computerised Decision Support System.
CDSU   : Communicable Diseases Surveillance Unit.
CDT   : Clock Drawing Test.
               Clostridium defficile Toxin.
CD4T   : Cluster of Differentiation 4 T-helper Lymphocytes.
CDU   : Chemical Dependence Unit.
               Clinical Decision Unit.

CE   : Capillary Electrolysis.
               Conformit`e European (Mark).
CEA   : Carcino-Embryonic Antigen. (Ref. an Immunochemistry marker).
               Carotid Endarterectomy.
               Caudal Extradural Analgesia.
               Clinical Excellence Awards.
               Continuous Epidural Analgesia.
               Cultured Epithelial Autografts.
CEACCP : Continuing Education in Anaesthesia, Critical Care and Pain.
CEB   : Caudal Epidural Block.
CED   :"Coverage with Evidence Development."(Ref. offers patients access to new treatments in USA; Europe; Canada; Australia).
CEI   : Committee for Ethical Issues in Medicine
               Continuous Epidural Infusion.
CEMACH : Confidential Enquiry into Maternal and Child Health.
CEMD   : Confidential Enquiry into Maternal Deaths.
CENSA   : Confederation of European National Societies of Anaesthesiologists.
CENTRA(L) : Cochrane Central Register of Controlled Trials.
CEOT   : Calcifying Epithelial Odontogenic Tumour.
CEPD   : Continuing Education and Professional Development.
CEPOD   : Confidential Enquiry in Post-operative Deaths.
CER   : Comparative Effectiveness Research.(Ref. compare benefits of competing drugs).

Control Event Rate.
Cost Effective Ratio.

CESPM : Council for Education in Pharmaceutical Medicine. (USA).

CESDI : Confidential Enquiry into Stillbirths and Deaths in Infancy.

CESR : Certificate for Eligibility for Specialist Registration.

CEX : Clinical Evaluation Exercise.

CF : Cardiac Failure.
Complement Fixation.
Cystic Fibrosis.

CFA : Complete Freud`s Adjuvant. (Ref. in Pain treatment)
Cryptogenic Fibrosis (or Fibrosing) Alveolitis.

CFAM : Cerebral Function Analysis Monitor.

CFD : Colour Flow Doppler.

CfH : Connecting for Health.

CFL : Calcaneofibular Ligament.

CFM : Cerebral Function Monitor.
Colour Flow Mapping.

CFRD : Cystic Fibrosis-related Diabetes.

CFS : Chronic Fatigue Syndrome. (Ref. see Myolagia Encephalomyelitis; **ME**).

CFT : Clot Formation Time.
Complement Fixation Test.

CFTR : Cystic Fibrosis Transmembrane Conductance Regulator (or Regulation).
Cystic Fibrosis Transmembrane Receptor.

CFU : Colony Forming Units. (Ref. to Bacterial load).

CG : Clinical Governance.
Clinical Guidelines.

CGA : Comprehensive Geriatric Assessment.

CGCG : Central Giant Cell Granuloma.

CGD : Chronic Granulomatous Disease.

Cgh : Cough.

CGIN : Cervical Glandular Intraepithelial Neoplasia.

CGL : Chronic Granulocytic Leukaemia.

CGMP : Cyclic Guanosine Monophosphate.
CGO : Common Gas Outlet. (Ref. Anaesthetic machine gas-mixture outlet).
CGRP : Calcitonin Gene-related Peptide.
CGST : Clinical Governance Support Team (of the **NHS**).
cGVHD : Chronic Graft-versus-Host Disease.

Ch : Child/Children/Chronic.
CH : Community Hospital.
CHAI : Commission for Healthcare Audit and Inspection (Healthcare Commission).
CHAQ : Childhood Health Assessment Questionnaire.
CHARGE : Coloboma, Heart defects, Choanal atresia, Retarded growth, Genital anomalies, Ear abnormalities.
CHARM : Candestarn in Heart Failure Assessment of Reduction in Mortality and Mobidity.
CHARMS : Cornwal Heart Attack Rehabilitation Management Study.
CHART : Continuous Hyperfractionated Accelerated Radiotherapy.
Ch.AT : Choline Acetyl Transferase.
CHB : Complete Heart Block.
Congenital Heart Block.
CHC : Combined Hormonal Contraception
Community Health Centre.
CHD : Congenital Heart Disease.
Coronary Heart Disease.
CHDA : Child Health, Development and Aging.
ChEI : Cholineesterase Inhibitor.
Chem. : Chemistry or Chemical.
CHEOPS : Children's Hospital of Eastern Ontario Pain Scale. (Canada).
CHF : Congestive Heart Failure.
Chronic Heart Failure.
CHFG : Clinical Human Factors Group.
CHI : Closed Head Injury.
Commission for Health Improvement.
Congenital Hearing Impairment
Creatinine Height Index.

CHIP	: Channel-forming Integral Protein.
CHIPPS	: Children and Infants Post-operative Pain Scale.
CHIQ	: Centre for Health Information Quality.
CHL	: Conductive Hearing Loss.
CHM	: Commission on Human Medicines.
CHMP	: Committee for Human Medicinal Products (for Human use). (USA).
CHMS	: Central Health and Miscellaneous Services.
CHO	: Carbohydrate.
Cho-vac	: Cholera Vaccine.
CHP	: Capsular Hydrostatic Pressure.
CHRPE	: Congenital Hypertrophy of Retinal Pigment Epithelium.
CHS	: Che`diak-Higashi Syndrome. (Ref. a rare autosomal recessive disorder).
CHTE	: Clinical Centre for Health Technology Evaluation.
C/I	: Contraindication.
CI	: Cardiac Index. Confidence Interval. Contraindicated.
CIsegmen	: Cervical Spine segment.
CIALP	: C-Immunoassay for Antigenic Latex Proteins.
CIC	: Circulating Immune Complex. Crisis Intervention Centre.
CICU	: Cardiac Intensive Care Unit.
CI-CV	: Can`t Intubate-Can`t Ventilate.
CIE	: Counter-current Immuno-electrophoresis.
CIE 1	: C 1-Esterase Inhibitor.
CIM	: Critical Illness Myopathy.
CIMP	: Clinical Information Management Programme.
CIN	: Cervical Intraepithelial Neoplasia. (Ref. in Gynaecology). Contrast Induced Nephropathy.
CIND	: Cognitive Impairment no Dementia.
CIOMS	: Council for International Organisations of Medical Sciences.
CIP	: Critical Illness Polyneuropathy.
Circ.	: Circulation/Circumcision.
CIS	: Carcinoma in situ. Corporate Indemnity Solution.

CIT : Clinical Information Technology.
Cognitive Impairment Test.

CJD : Creutzfeldt-Jakob Disease.

CK : Creatinine Kinase
CK-MB : Creatinine Kinase-Myocardial Isoenzyme B.

Cl : Chloride.
CL : Cleft Lip.
CLs : Clinical Lectureships.
CLAPA : Cleft Lip and Palate Association.
CLBP : Chronic Lower Back Pain.
CLD : Chronic Lung Disease.
CLDP : Chronic Lung Disease of Prematurity.
CLDT : Community Learning Difficulties Team.
CLEA : Continuous Labour Epidural Analgesia.
CLI : Critical Limb Ischaemia.
CLIA : Clinical Laboratories Improvement Act (1988). (USA).
CLL : Chronic Lymphocytic Leukaemia.
CLM : Cutaneous Larva Migrans.
CLMA : Classic Laryngeal Mask Airway.
CLO : Campylobacter-like Organism. (Ref. a rapid Urea test).
Columnar-lined Oesophagus; (Barrett`s).
CLP : Caecal Ligation and Perfusion.
Cleft Lip and Palate.
CLT : Chronic Lymphocytic Thyroiditis.
CLVM : Complex Combined Vascular Malformation.

Cm : Centimetre.
CM : Case or Care Manager.
Cryptococcal Meningitis.
CMAPs : Compound (Motor) Muscle-Action Potential.
CMC : Carpo-Metacarpal.
CMCJ : Carpo-Metacarpal Joint.
CMD : Congenital Muscular Dystrophy.
Count Median Diameter. (Ref. particle size in Anaesthetic circuits).

	Craniomandibular Dysfunction.
CME	: Continuing Medical Education.
CMEC	: Central Mucoepidermoid Carcinoma.
CMF	: Cyclophosphamide, Methotrexate, 5–Fluorouracil.
CMG	: Compressomyography.(Ref. a new neuromuscular transmission monitor).
	Current Medicine Group.
CMHT	: Community Mental Health Team.
CML	: Chronic Myeloid Leukaemia.
CMML	: Chronic Myelomonocytic Leukaemia.
CMN	: Congenital Melanocytic Nevus (or Nevi).
CMO	: Chief Medical Officer.
CMOS	: Complementary Metal Oxide Semiconductors. (Ref. Solid State Sensors).
CMP	: Case Mix Programme.
	Clinical Management Plan.
CMR	: Cerebral Metabolic Rate.
	Cardiovascular Magnetic Resonance.
CMRO₂	: Cerebral Metabolic Rate for Oxygen.
CMT	: Clinical Midwife Teacher.
	Combined Movement Therapy.
	Core Medical Training.
CMV	: Continuous Mandatory Ventilation.
	Controlled Mandatory Ventilation.
	Conventional Mechanical Ventilation.
	Cytomegalovirus.
CMVP	: Cytomegaloviral Pneumonia.
CN	: Central Nerve. (USA).
	Cranial Nerve
CNAP	: Compound Nerve Action Potential.
CNB	: Central Neuraxial Nerve Block (or Blockade).
CNEP	: Continous Negative Extrathoracic Pressure.
CNG	: Community Nutrition Group.
CNO	: Chief Nursing Officer.
CNP	: C-type Natriuretic Peptide. (Ref. in cardiac failure).
CNS	: Central Nervous System.
	Clinical Negligence Scheme for Trusts.

Clinical Nurse Specialist.

Co	: Cobalt.
	Coccygeal.
C/O(c/o)	: Complain of (or Complaining of).
CO	: Carbon Monoxide.
	Cardiac Output.
	Casualty Officer.
CO2	: Carbon Dioxide.
COA (CoA)	: Coarctation of the Aorta.
COAD	: Chronic Obstructive Airway Disease.
COC	: Combined Oral Contraception.
COCP	: Combined Oral Contraception Pill.
COETT	: Cuffed Oral Endotracheal Tube.
COFHP	: Chronic Oral, Facial, Head Pain.
COHb	: Carboxyhaemoglobin.
COHSE	: Confederation of Health Service Employees.
COG	: Centre of Gravity.
COLD	: Chronic Obstructive Lung Disease.
COM	: Centre of Mass.
COMA	: Committee On Medical Aspects (of Food and Nutrition Policy).
COMARE	: Committee on Medical Aspects of Radiation in the Environment.
COME	: Chronic Otitis Media with Effusion.
COMEAP	: Committee on the Medical Aspects of Air Pollutants.
COMET	: Comparative Obstetric Mobile Epidural Trial.
COMFA	: Comparative Molecular Field Analysis.(Ref. in **i.v.** Anaesthesia).
COMP	: Committee on Orphan Medicinal Products. (USA).
COMPANION	: Comparison of Medical Therapy, Pacing and Defibrillation.
COMT	: Catechol-O-Methyl Transferase.
Con.	: Consultant.
CONS	: Coagulase-Negative Staphylococci,
CONSORT	: Consolidated Standards of Reporting Trials (1996–2010).
CO	: Cardiac Output.

		Carbon Monoxide.
CO2	:	Carbon Dioxide.
COOP	:	Care of Old People.
COP	:	Centre of Pressure.
		Change of Plaster.
		Colloid Oncotic Pressure.
		Colloid Osmotic Pressure.
COPA	:	Cuffed Oropharyngeal Airway. (Ref. an Anaesthetic Device).
COPE	:	Committee on Publication Ethics.
COPES	:	Community Oriented Programme Environment Scale.
		Crisis-Oriented Personal Evaluation Scale.
COPC	:	Community-Oriented Primary Care.
COPD	:	Chronic Obstructive Pulmonary Disease.
COPERNICUS	:	Carvedil O1 Prospective Randomized Cumulative Survival (Trial).
COPMED	:	Conference of Postgraduate Medical Deans.
COR	:	Cervico-Ocular Reflex.
		Conditioned-Orientation Reflex.
COREC	:	Central Oxford Research Ethics Committee.
CO2R	:	Carbon Dioxide Reactivity.
COSHH	:	Control of Substances Hazardous to Health.
COSTR	:	Consesus On Science and Treatment Recommendations.
COXs	:	Cyclo-Oxygenases.
COX-2	:	Cyclo-Oxygenase 2.
COXIs	:	Cyclo-Oxygenase Inhibitors.
C`p	:	Chickenpox.
CP	:	Carbamide Peroxide.
		Cardiopulmonary.
		Centralized Procedure. (USA).
		Cerebral Palsy.
		Cicatricial Pemphigoid.
		Cleft Palate.
		Community Practitioner.
CPA	:	Care Programme Approach.
		Cerebral-Pointing Angle.
		Colour Power Angiography.

Criminal Procedures Act.

Cyproterone Acetate.

CPAP : Continuous Positive Airway Pressure.

CP-50 : Plasma Concentration to prevent response in 50% of subjects.

CPB : Cardio-Pulmonary Bypass.

CPCs : Cerebral Performance Categories. (Ref. Glasgow Score).

CPD : Calcium Phosphate Deposition.

Cephalo-Pelvic Disproportion.

Cognitive Behavioural Therapy.

Continuing Professional Development.

CPEP : Calcium for Pre-eclampsia Prevention (Trial).

CPET : Cardiopulmonary Exercise Testing.

CPH : Certificate of Public Health.

Clinical Centre for Public Health Excellence.

CPI : Continous Process Improvement. (USA).

CPK : Creatinine Phosphokinase.

CPM : Continuous Passive Motion.(Ref. analgesia after Total Knee Replacement.)

CPMP : Committee on Proprietary Medicinal Products. (USA).

Central Protein Myelinolysis.(Ref. neurodemyelination and hyponatraemia).

CPN : Community Psychiatric Nurse.

CPNB : Continuous Peripheral Nerve Block.

CPOE : Computerised Physician (Provider) Order Entry.

CPP(e-CPP) : Cerebral Perfusion Pressure (estimated.)

CPP : Calcium Pyrophosphate.

Cerebral Perfusion Pressure.

Certificate of a Pharmaceutical Product.

Chronic Pelvic Pain.

Clinical Portal Project. (Ref. access to patients records).

Coronary Perfusion Pressure.

CPPC : Calcium Pyrophosphate Crystals.

CPPD : Calcium Phosphate Dihydrate.

CPPIH : Commission for Patients and Public Involvement in Health.

CPR : Cardiopulmonary Resuscitation.

Child Protection Register.

CPSM	: Council for Professions Supplementary to Medicine.
CPT	: Carnitine-Palmity Transferase.
	Chest Physiotherapy.
CPX	: Cardiopulmonary Exercise Testing.(Ref. sometimes referred to as **CPET**).
CQC	: Care Quality Commission.
CQI	: Continuous Quality Improvement. (USA).
CQUIN	: Commissioning for Quality and Innovation Payment Framework.(Ref. to Quality improvement in the **NHS**).
CR (Cr)	: Chromium.
	Creatinine.
CRA	: Continuous Regional Analgesia.
CrAg	: Cryptococcal Antigen.
CRAG	: Clinical Resource Audit Group.
CRAMS	: Circulation, Respiration, Abdomen, Motor, Speech (Scoring).
CRB	: Criminal Records Bureau.
CRBD	: Catheter-Related Bladder Discomfort.
CRC	: Cancer Research Campaign.
	Cancer Research Centre.
	Colorectal Cancer.
CRCO₂	: Cerebral Vascular Reactivity to Carbon Dioxide.
CRD	: Centre for Research and Dissemination (of the **NHS**).
CRDIQ	: Chronic Respiratory Disease Index Questionnaire.
CRE	: Care Record Elements.
CREST	: Calcinosis, Raynaud phenomenon, Oesophageal involvement, Sclerodactyl, Telangiectasia (Syndrome).
CRF	: Case Report Form. (USA).
	Chronic Renal Failure.
	Clinical Research Facility.
	Corticotrophin-releasing Factor.
CRH	: Corticotrophin Releasing Hormone.
CRHP	: Council for Regulation of Healthcare Professionals.
CRIB	: Clinical Risk Index for Babies.
CRL	: Crown Rump Length (of Foetus).
CRM	: Committee on the Review of Medicines.

	Crisis Resource Management (Behaviour):(Ref. to performance scoring).
CRMF	: Cancer Relief Macmillan Fund.
CRMO	: Chronic Recurrent Multifocal Osteomyelitis.
CRP	: Canalith Repositioning Procedure.
	C-Reactive Protein. (Ref. inflammatory biochemical marker).
CRPP	: Closed Reduction and Percutaneous Pin (fixation).
CRPS	: Complex Regional Pain Syndrome.(or Chronic Regional Pain Syndrome).
	Council of the Royal Pharmaceutical Society.
CRQs	: Contract Research Organisations.
CRRT	: Continuous Renal Replacement Therapy.
CRS	: Care Records Service.
	Compliance of the Respiratory System.
	Cough Receptor Sensitivity.
CRT	: Capillary Refill Time.
	Cardiac Resynchronisation Therapy.
CRU	: Coronary Rehabilitation Unit.
Cryo	: Cryoglobulinemia.
CS	: Caesarean Section.
	Cardiac Sphincter.
	Clinical Science.
	Compartment Syndrome.
	Coronary Sinus.
CSgas	: Chlorobenzylidine Malononitrile (gas).
C & S	: Circulation and Sensation.
	Culture and Sensitivity.
CSA	: Child Sexual Abuse.
	Compressed Spectral Assay.
	Continuous Subarachnoid (or Spinal) Anaesthesia.
	Cross-Sectional Area. (Ref. in Transoesophageal Echocardiography).
CSII	: Continuous Subcutaneous Insulin Infusion.
CSAG	: Clinical Standards Advisory Group.
CSAR	: Conservative Subtraction-Addition Rhinoplasty.
CSBS	: Clinical Standards Board for Scotland.

CSD	: Committee on Safety of Drugs.
CSE	: Combined Spinal Epidural.
	Council of Science Editors.
CSF	: Cerebral Spinal Fluid.
	Colon-Stimulating Factor.
CSHT	: Context-Sensitive Half-Time.(Ref. time for i.v
	Anaesthetic drug concentration to fall by 50% of the
	original concentration).
CSI	: Cerebral State Index.
CSIP	: Care Services Improvement Partnership.
CSL	: Commissioning Support for London.
CSM	: Carotid Sinus Massage.
	Cerebral State Minitor.(Ref. monitoring of depth of
	General Anaesthesia).
	Committee on Safety of Medicines. (Ref. now under
	CHM).
CSOM	: Chronic Suppurative Otitis Media.
CSP	: Chartered Society of Physiotherapists.
CSS	: Carotid Sinus Syndrome.
	Churg-Strauss Syndrome.
	Council for Science and Society.
CSSD	: Central Sterilisation Service Department.
CST	: Clinical Skills Trainer.
CSU	: Catheter Specimen of Urine.
CSV	: Computerised Systems Validation.
CSWS	: Cerebral Salt-Wasting Syndrome.
CT	: Calcitonin.
	Computed (Computerized)Tomography.
	Core Training (or Trainee).
CTA	: Clinical Trials Authorization. (USA).
CTC	: Clinical Trials Certification. (USA).
CTCL	: Cuteneous T-Cell Lymphoma.
CTD	: Common Technical Document. (USA).
	Connective Tissue Disease.
CTG	: Cardiotocography (or Cardiotocogram.).(Ref.
	monitoring in Obstetrics).
CTIMPs	: Clinical Trials of Investigational Medicinal Products.
CTL	: Cytotoxic T-cell.

CTO	: Compulsory Treatment Order.
	Community Treatment Order.
CTPA	: Computerized Tomography(**CT**) Pulmonary Angiogram.
CTS	: Carpal Tunnel Syndrome.
CTSIB	: Clinical Test of Sensory Integration on Balance.
CTT	: Colonic Transit Time.
CTX	: Clinical Trials Exemption. (USA).
	Cross-linked C-Telepeptide.
Cu	: Copper.
CUC	: Chronic Ulcerative Colitis.
CUE	: Confidential Unit Exclusion. (Ref. Bloood Transfusion in the USA).
CUS	: Catheter Urine Sample.
CV	: Cardiovascular.
	Central-Venous.
	Coefficient of Variance.
	Curriculum Vitae.
CVA	: Cerebral Vascular Accident.
CVC	: Central Venous Catheter.
CVD	: Cardiovascular Disease.
CVI	: Chronic Venous Insufficiency.
CVP	: Cell Volume Profile.
	Central Venous Pressure.
CVE	: Cerebral Vascular Episode (or Event).
CVOs	: Circumventricular Organs.
CVS	: Cardiovascular System.
	Chorionic Villus Sampling.
CVT	: Cerebral Veinous Thrombosis.
CVVHF	: Continuous Veno-Venous Haemofiltration.
Cx	: Cervix.
CX	: Circumflex Coronary Artery.
CXR	: Chest X-ray.
CWD	: Consistent with Dates.
CWP	: Coal Workers Pneumoconiosis.

CW/R	: Consultant Ward Round.
CyA	: Cyclosporin A.
CYP	: Cytochrome P450 (Isoenzyme).
CZ	: Coryza.
d.	: Day/s.
	Density.
D	: Decreased.
	Diagnosis.
D2	: Ergocalciferol.
D3	: Cholecalciferol.
DA	: Dental Anaesthetic.
	Dietetic Assistant.
	Diploma in Anaesthesia.
	Dopamine.
DAFNE	: Dose Adjustment for Normal Eating (Programme).
DAI	: Diffuse Axonal Injury. (Ref. Neuro-damage).
DALI	: Dartmouth Assessment of Life Style Instrument.
DALY	: Disability Adjusted Life Years.
DAPE	: Data, Assessment, Plan, Education.
DAPRE	: Daily Adjustable Progressive Resistive Exercise (Technique).
DARD	: Dyspnoea-Associated Respiratory Distress.
DARE	: Data,Action,Response,Education. (Ref. Database of Reviews of Effectiveness).
DART	: Development for Anti-Retroviral Therapy.
DAS	: Difficult Airway Society.
	Disease Assessment Score.
DASH	: Dietary Approaches to Stop Hypertension.
	Disabilities of Arm, Shoulder, and Hand.
DASS	: Depression, Anxiety, Stress Scale.
DAT	: Dementia of the Alzheimer Type.
	Diet as Tolerated.
	Direct Antiglobulin (Antigen) Test. (USA).
	Drug Action Team.

DBCP : Dibromochloropropane.
DBP (dBP) : Diastolic Blodd Pressure.
DBS : Double-Burst Stimulation.
Deep Brain Stimulation.
DBT : Dialectical Behavioural Therapy.
Dry Bulb Temperature.(Ref. measure of Environment Temperature load).

DC : Dental Clinic.
Diabetic Clinic.
Dichorionic (Twins).
Direct Current.
D/C : Discontinue.
D&C : Dilatation and Curettage.
DCA : Day Clinic Association. (USA).
: Directional Coronary Atherectomy.
D&E : Dilatation and Evacuation.
DCI : Ductal Carcinoma in situ.
DCCT : Diabetic Control and Complications Trial.
DCD : Developmental Co-ordination Disorder.
Diploma of Child Development.
DCE : Dynamic Constant External Resistance (Exercise).
DCH : Diploma in Child Health.
DCIA : Deep Circumflex Iliac Artery.
DCIS : Ductal Carcinoma in situ.
DCIV : Deep Circumflex Iliac Vein.
DCL-Hb : Diaspirin Cross-linked Haemoglobin.
DCM : Dilated Cardiomyopathy.
DCO : Damage Control Orthopaedics.
DCP : Dynamic Compression Plate.
DCR : Dacro-Cysto—Rhinostomy.
DCRT : Disease-Controlling Rheumatic Therapy; (or Rheumatic Drugs).
DCS : Dynamic Compression Screw.
DCT : Direct Coomb`s Test.
Distal Convoluted Tubule. (Ref. of the Kidneys).

DD : Delta Down. (Ref. in Volaemia.)

	Differential Diagnosis.
DDA	: Dispensing Doctors Association.
	Dangerous Drugs Act.
DDAVP	: Desamino-8-D-arginine Vasopressin (or Desmopressin).
DDC	: Zalcitabine. (Ref. Reverse Transcriptase Inhibitor in treatment of **AIDS**).
DDH	: Developmental Dysplasia of the Hip.
DDI	: Didanosine. (Ref. Reverse Transcriptase Inhibitor in **AIDS** treatment).
DDM	: Diploma in Dermatological Medicine.
DDMAC	: Division of Drug Marketing, Advertising and Communications. (USA).
DDRB	: Doctors and Dentists Review Body.
DDSRCS	: Doctorate in Dental Surgery, Royal College of Surgeons.
DDT	: Dichlorodiphenyl Trichloroethane.

DEBRA	: Dystrophic Epidermolysis Bullosa Research Association.
DEC	: Diethylcarbamazine
DED	: Date Expected Delivery.
DEFRA	: Department for Environment, Food, and Rural Affairs.
DEJ	: Dermal-Epidermal Junction.
DEN	: District Enrolled Nurse.
DENT	: Dental Exposure Normalisation Technique.
DEO	: Disability Employment Officer.
DERM	: Dermatology.
DES	: Dietary Energy Supply.
	Diethylstilbestrol.
	Directed Enhanced Service.(Ref. for patients with learning disabilities).
	Drug-eluting Stent.
DESMOND	: Diabetes Education Self-Managed Ongoing and Newly Diagnosed (Programme).
DEX	: Dexmedetomide. (Ref. a new analgesic agent).
DEXA	: Dual-Energy X-ray Absorptiometry; (or Dual Emission X-ray Absorptiometry).
DF	: Dermatofibroma.
	Fractal Dimension. (Ref. in the analysis of **HRV**).
DFA	: Direct Fluorescent Antibody.

DFDBA   : Demineralised Freeze-dried Bone Allograft.
                    Decalcified Freeze-dried Bone Allograft.
DFES (DfES): Department for Education and Skills.
DFP   : Diastolic Filling Period.
DFSP   : Dermatofibrosarcoma Protuberans.

DGH   : District General Hospital.
DGI   : Disseminated Gonococcal Infection.

Dh   : Dermatitis hypertiformis.
DH   : Day Hospital.
                    Dermatitis Herpetiformis.
                    Department of Health. (see **DoH**).
                    Drug History.
DHA   : Docosahexaenoic Acid.
DHCA   : Deep Hypothermic Circulatory Arrest.
DHCC   : Dihydroxycholecalciferol.
DHCP   : Dental Healthcare Provider.
DHEA   : Dehydroepiandrosterone.
DHEA-S (DHAS): Dehydroepiandrosterone-Sulphate.
DHF   : Dengue Haemorrhagic Fever.
DHI   : Dynamic Hyper-Inflation.
DHS   : Dynamic Hip Screw.
DHSS   : Department of Health and Social Security.
DHSSPS : Department of Health,Social Services and Public Safety.
                    (Northern Ireland).
DHT   : Dihydrotestosterone.

DI   : Diabetes Inspidus.
                    Donor Insemination.
                    Detrusor Instability.
DIA   : Diaphragm.
                    Drug Information Association. (USA).
DIB   : Difficulty in Breathing.
DIC   : Died in Casualty.
                    Disseminated Intravascular Coagulation; (or
                    Disseminating Intravascular Coagulopathy).
DICOM   : Digital Imaging and Communications in Medicine.

DIDMOAD : Diabetes Inspidus, Diabetes Mellitus, Optic Atrophy, and Deafness.
DIF : Direct Immunofluorescence.
DIG : Digitalis Investigation Group (Study).
DIMS : Disorders of Initiating and Maintaining Sleep.
DIP : Distal Interphalangeal.
DIPJ : Distal Interphalangeal Joint.
Desquamative Interstitial Pneumonia.
DipN : Diploma in Nursing.
DISCUS : Dyskinesia Identification System-Condensed User Scale.
DISH : Diffuse Idiopathic Skeletal Hyperostosis.
DIT : Dietary Induced Thermogenesis.
Diidotyrosine.

DJ : Duodeno-Jejunal.
DJD : Degenerative Joint Disease.
DJF : Duodenojejunal-Flexure.

DKA : Diabetic Keto-acidosis.
dL : Decilitre.
DL : Diagnostic Laparoscopy.
Diagnostic Laparotomy.
Direct Laryngoscopy.
DLA : Disability Living Allowance.
DLB : Dementia with Lewy Bodies.
DLCO : Diffusion Lung Carbon Monoxide. (Ref. Lung function test in Lung Surgery).
DLE : Desseminated Lupus Erythematosus.
Discoid Lupus Erythematosus.
DLEBT : Double Lumen Endo-bronchial Tube.
DLF : Disabled Living Foundation.
DLI : Donor Leucocyte Infusion.
DLT : Double Lumen Tube.

DM : Dermatomyositis.
Diabetes Mellitus.
DM2 : Diabetes Mellitus (Type 2).
DMAC : Disseminated Mycobacterium Avium Complex.

DMARDs	: Disease-modifying Anti-Rheumatic Drugs.
DMB	: Demineralised Bone.
DMD	: Disease Modifying Drugs.
	Duchenne Muscular Dystrophy.
DMEM	: Dulbecco`s Modified Eagles Medium.
DMF	: Decayed, Missing, Filled.
dmft	: Decayed Missing and Filled Teeth. (Deciduous teeth).
DMFT	: Decayed Missing and Filled Teeth (Permanent teeth).
DML	: Distal Motor Latency.
DMPA	: Depot Medroxyprogestrone Acetate.
DMS	: Defence Medical Services.
DMSA	: Dimercaptosuccinic Acid.(Ref. Technetium isotope used in scanning children with Hypertension).
DMST	: Dexamethasone Suppression Test.
DMT	: Dimethyltryptamine.
DN	: Diploma in Nursing.
	District Nurse.
DNA	: Deoxyribo-Nucleic Acid.
	Did Not Attend.
	District Nursing Association.
DNAR	: Do Not Attempt Resuscitation.
DNE(DipNEd)	: Diploma in Nursing Education.
DNKA	: Did Not Keep Appointment.
DNM	: Descending Necrotising Mediastinitis.
DNR	: Do Not Resuscitate.
DNS	: Deflected Nasal Septum.
DNSG	: Diabetes and Nutrition Study Group.
DNT	: District Nurse Teacher.
DO	: Direct Oesophagoscopy.
DOA	: Depth of Anaesthesia.
	Dead on Arrival.
DOB(DoB)	: Date of Birth.
DOC	: Deoxycorticosterone.
	Dynamic Orthotic Cranioplasty.
DOES	: Disorders of Excessive Somnolence.
DoH (DH)	: Department of Health.

DOM	: Department of Medicine.
DOMS	: Delayed-onset of Muscle Soreness.
DOPAC	: (3,4) Dihydroxyphenylacetic Acid.
DOPR	: Delta Opioid Receptor.
DOPS	: Direct Observation of Procedural Skill. (Ref. Video Laryngoscopy).
DOS	: Department of Surgery.
	Diffuse Oesophageal Spasm.
DOT	: Directly Observed Therapy (or Treatment)
DOTS	: Directly Observed Therapy Shortcourse.
DP	: Dental Plate.
	Direct Pharyngoscopy.
DPA	: Data Protection Act 1998 (U.K)
	Descending Palatine Artery.
DPB	: Dental Practice Board.
DPD	: Drug Policy Division.
	Dysgenetic Polycystic Disease.
DPF	: Dental Practitioner`s Formulary.
DPG (2-3 DPG):	(2-3) Dihydrophospho-Gluconase.
	Diphosphoglycerate.
DPH	: Department of Public Health.
	Diploma in Public Health.
	Director of Public Health.
DPLD	: Diffuse Parenchymal Lung Disease.
DPM	: Diploma in Psychological Medicine.
DPMD	: Defence Postgraduate Medical Deanery.
DPP	: Delta Pulse Pressure.
DPR	: Data Protection Register.
DPS	: Design for Patients Safety. (Ref. Helen Haulyn Centre at Royal College of Art).
	Diversified Pharmaceutical Services. (USA).
DPT	: Diphtheria, Pertussis, Tetanus.
Dr	: Doctor.
DR	: Detection rate.
	Diabetic Retinopathy.
	Doctor.

DRCOG : Diploma of the Royal College of Obstetrics and Gynaecology.

DRE : Digital Rectal Examination.

DREZ : Dorsal Root Entry Zone.

DRG : Diagnosis Related Group. (Ref. Hospital Admissions records).
Dorsal Root Ganglion. (Ref. of Central Nervous System).

DRLs : Dose Reference Levels. (Ref. in medical radiodiagnostic practices).

DRPLA : Detanto-Rubro-Pallido-Luysian Atrophy.

DRPs : Drag-reducing Polymers.

DRUJ : Distal Radio-ulnar Joint.

DRV : Dietary Reference Value.

DRVVT : Dilute Russell`s Viper Venom Time.

DS : Day Surgery.
Disseminated Sclerosis.
Double Strength.
Down`s Syndrome.

DSA : Digital Subtraction Angiography.

dsDNA : Double-stranded **DNA.**

DSE : Dobutamine Stress Echocardiography.

Dsg : Desmoglein.

DSH : Deliberate Self-harm.

DSM : Diagnostic and Statistical Manual (of Mental Disorders).

DSM-IV-TR : Diagnostic and Statistical Manual of Mental Disorders.

DSPD : Dangerous and Severe Personality Disorder.

DSPS : Delayed Sleep-phase Syndrome.(Ref. one syndrome of sleep disorders).

DSS : Decision Support System.
Dejeriue-Sottas Syndrome. (Ref. hereditary motor-sensory neuropathy).
Dengue Shock Syndrome.
Department of Social Security.

DSST : Digit Symbol Substitution Test. (Ref. a measure of cognitive function).

DST : Dexamethasone Suppression Test.

DSU : Day Surgery Unit.

Drug Safety Update.

DT	: Deceleration Time.
	Delirium Tremens.
	Diphtheria and Tetanus (Toxoids).
	Drainage Tube.
DTs	: Delirium Tremens.
DTB	: Drugs and Therapeutics Bulletin.
DTC	: Diagnosis and Treatment Centre.
	Direct to Consumer (Advertising). (USA).
	Donor Transplant Co-ordinator.
DTCA	: Direct to Consumer Advertising (Campaigns). (USA).
DTM&H	: Diploma in Tropical Medicine and Hygiene.
DTN	: Diphtheria Toxin Normal.
DTP	: Diptheria, Tetanus and Pertussis.
DTPA	: Diethelene-Triamine-Penta-Acetic Acid (Technetium isotope).
DTS	: Dipyridamole-Thallium Scintigraphy.
DU	: Duodenal Ulcer.
DUB	: Dysfunctional Uterine Bleeding.
DURs	: Drug Utilisation Reviews. (USA).
DUS	: Duplex Ultrasound (of the Carotid).
DV	: Domiciliary Visit.
D & V	: Diarrhoea and Vomiting.
DVA	: Dynamic Visual Acuity.
DVT	: Deep Vein Thrombosis.
D/W (d/w)	: Discussed with.
DWI	: Diffusion Weighted Imaging.
DWS	: Dorsal Wrist Syndrome.
DXA	: Dual-energy X-Ray Absorptiometry (Scanning.): (Ref. in Osteoporosis diagnosis and management; also see under **DEXA**).
DXT	: Deep X-ray Therapy; (or Deep Radiotherapy).

Dysm : Dysmenorrhoea.

Dz : Disease.
DZ : Dizygous or Dizygotic (Twins).

E : Epigastric.
E 3 : Oestriol.
EA : Enteropathic Arthritis.
EAA : Essential Amino Acids.
   European Academy of Anaesthesiologists.
   Extrinsic Allergic Alveolitis.
EAATs : Excitatory Amino Acid Transporters.
EABV : Effective Arterial Blood Volume.
EAC : External Auditory Canal.
EACA : Epsilon Amino-caproic Acid.
EAEC : Entero-Aggregative Escherichia. Coli.
EAP : Endoscopic Access Port.
EAR : Estimated Average (Nutritional) Requirement.
EARR : External Apical Root Resorption.
EAM : External Auditory Meatus.
EASI : Employment Agency Standards Inspectorate. (Ref. a
   regulator of Employment Agencies).
EASL : European Association for the Study of the Liver.
EAT : Ectopic Atrial Tachycardia.

EBA : Electron Beam Angiography.
   Epidermolysis Bullosa Acquisita.
   Ethoxybenzoic Acid.
EBD : Evidence-Based Dentistry.
EBH : Evidence-Based Healthcare.
EBHC : Evidence-Based Health Care.
EBL : Endemic Burkitt Lymphoma.
EBLL : Elevated Blood Lead Level.
EBM : Evidence-Based Medicine.
   Expressed Breast Milk.
EBMH : Evidence-Based Mental Health.
EBP : Epidural Blood Patch.
   Evidence-Based Practice.

EBS	: Emergency Bed Service.
EBT	: Electron Beam Tomography.
EBV	: Epstein-Barr Virus.
e/c	: Enteric-coated.
EC	: Emergency Contraception.
ECs	: Endothelial Cells.
ECA	: Epidemiological Catchment Area.
	External Carotid Artery.
ECASS	: European Cooperative Acute Stroke Study.
ECC	: Emergency Care Centre.
ECD	: European Centre for Disease Prevention and Control.
ECE	: Endothelial Converting Enzyme.
ECF	: Epirubicin; Cisplatin and 5–Fluorouracil.
	Extended Care Facility.
	Extracellular Fluid.
ECG	: Electrocardiogram.
ECHO	: Echocardiography.
	Economic Clinical and Humanistic Outcomes. (USA).
	Entero-Cytopathogenic Human Orphan (Virus).
ECM	: External Cardiac Massage.
	Extracellular Matrix.
ECMDs	: European Confederation of Medical Devices.
ECMO	: Extra-corporeal Membrane Oxygenation.
ECR	: Extra-Contractual Referral.
ECRS	: Empathy Construct Rating Scale.
ECS	: Endocervical Swab.
	Extra-Cellular Space.
ECST	: European Carotid Surgery Trial.
ECT	: Electro-Convulsive Therapy.
ECTD	: European Clinical Trials Directive.
ECV	: Effective Circulating Volume.
	External Cephalic Version.
ED	: Emergency Department. (Ref. Accident and Emegency See under **A & E**).
	Entropy Difference.
	Erectile Dysfunction.

	Every Day.
ED50	: Effective Dose to 50% of subjects.
EDA	: End-diastolic Area.
EDC	: Equality and Diversity Committee.
	Expected Date of Confinement.
EDD	: Expected Date of Delivery.
	Extended Daily Dialysis.
EDE	: Eating Disorders Examination.
EDF	: End Diasatolic Flow.
EDH	: Extra-Dural Haematoma.
EDHF	: Endothelium-derived Hyperpolarised Factor.
EDIC	: Epidemiology of Diabetes Interventions and Complications.
EDJ	: Enamel-Dentine Junction.
EDM	: Early Day Motion. (Ref. to commercialisation in the **NHS.**)
	Earl y Diastolic Murmur.
EDNOS	: Eating Disorder Not Otherwise Specified.
EDS	: Ehlers-Danlos Syndrome.
EDSS	: Expanded Disability Status Scale (or Scores.)
EDTA	: Ethylenediaminetetra-acetate. (Ref. in Laboratory blood specimens.)
	European Dialysis and Transplant Association.
EDV	: End-Diastolic Volume.
EE	: Energy Expenditure.
	Ethinyloestradiol.
EEA	: End-to-End Anastomosis.
EED	: Erythema Elevatum Diutinum.
EEG	: Electro-Encephalogram.
EEGR	: Electro-Encephalographic Response.
EENT	: Eyes, Ears, Nose, and Throat.
EEP	: End Expiratory Pressure.
EER	: Experimental Event Rate.
EF	: Ejection Fraction.
EFAs	: Essential Fatty Acids.
EFAD	: European Federation of the Associations of Dietitians.

EFM	: Electronic Foetal Monitoring (of the Heart).
EFL	: Epidural for Labour.
	External Financing Limit.
EFS	: European Food Safety Authority.
EFW	: Estimated Foetal Weight.

EG	: Ethylene Glycol.
EGC	: Early Gastric Ulcer.
EGF	: Epidermal Growth Factor.
EGFR	: Epidermal Growth Factor Receptor.
EGR	: Erythrocyte Glutathione Reductase.
EGRA	: Erythrocyte Glutathione Reductase Activity (Coefficient)

EHEC	: Entero-Haemorrhagic Escherichia. Coli.
EHOs	: Environmental Health Officers.
EHR	: Electronic Health Record.
EHRC	: Ethics in Human Research Committee.

EIA	: Enzyme Immuno-Assay.
EICP	: Early Impairment Cerebral Palsy.
EIEC	: Entero-Invasive Escherichia. Coli.
EIOC	: Effective Inspired Oxygen Concentration.
EIT	: Electrical Impedance Tomography.

EJV	: External Jugular Vein.

EKG	: Electrocardiogram. (USA).

EL	: Echo-graphic Level. (Ref. ultrasound-guided inter-vertebral epidural level).
ELBW	: Extremely Low Birth Weight.
ELCAP	: Early Lung Cancer Action Project. (Ref. Epidemiology of Lung cancers).
ELD	: End-Stage Liver Disease.
ELECTRA	: East London Randomised Trial for High Risk Asthma.
ELISA	: Enzyme-Linked Immunosorbent Assay. (Ref. Microbial Proteins and Antibodies detection Test).
ELND	: Elective Lymph Node Dissection.

EM	: Electron Microscopy.
	Emergency Medicine. (Ref. Accident and Emergency, **A& E,** Medicine).
	Erythema Migrans.
	Erythema Multiforme.
	Extensive Metaboliser.
EMA	: Endomysial Antibodies.
	European Medicines Agency.
EMAC	: Effective Management of Anaesthetic Crisises.
EMBASE	: European Electronic Database of Health-related Scientific References.
EMC	: Electromagnetic Compatibility.
EMCDDA	: European Monitoring Centre for Drugs and Drug Addiction.
EMD	: Electromechanical Dissociation.(Ref. Pulseless Electrical Activity; **PEA**).
	Enamel Matrix Derivative.
EMDP	: Extended Medical Degree Programme.
EMDR	: Eye Movement Desensitisation and Reprocessing.
EME	: Electrical Medical Engineers.
EMEA	: European Medicines Evaluation Agency.
EMF	: Endomyocardial Fibrosis.
EMG	: Electromyelogram.
	Electromyogram.
	Electromyographic (Activity). (Ref. monitoring depth of Anaesthesia).
EMI	: Elderly Mentally Infirm.
	Electromagnetic Interference.
EMID	: Environmentally Mediated Intellectual Decline.
EMIS	: Egton Medical Information System.
EMIT	: Enzyme Multiplied Immunoassay Technique.
EMLA	: Euteric Mixture of Local Anaesthetics (Lignocaine and Prilocaine **LA**).
EMO	: Esterase-Metabolised *u*-Opioid (Receptor Agonist.)
EMQ	: Extended Matching Question.
EMR	: Embryonic Mammary Ridge; (or the Milk line).
EMRS	: Emergency Medical Retrieval Service.

EMRSA	: Epidemic Methicillin-Resistant Staphylococcus Aureus (**MRSA**).
EMS	: Early Morning Stiffness.
	Emergency Medical Service.
EMTL	: Emergency Medicine, Trauma and Locomotion.
EMU	: Early Morning Urine (specimen).
EMW	: Early Morning Wakening.
EMWA	: European Medical Writers Association.
EN	: Enrolled Nurse.
	Enteral Nutrition.
ENA	: Extractable Nuclear Antigen.
ENaC	: Epithelial Sodium Channel.
ENB	: English National Board (for Nursing, Midwifery and Health Visiting).
	Esthesio-Neuro-Blastoma.
ENG	: Electronystagmography.
	Enrolled Nurse General.
ENL	: Erythema Nodosum Leprosum.
EN(M)	: Enrolled Nurse (Mental).
EN(MH)	: Enrolled Nurse (Mental Handicap).(Ref. now under Learning Disability).
ENP	: Emergency Nurse Practitioner.
ENT	: Ear, Nose and Throat.
ENTOG	: European Network of Trainees in Obstetrics and Gynaecology.
EO	: Extra-oral.
EOC	: Ease of Care.
	Epithelial Ovarian Cancer.
EOG	: Electro-Oculo-gram.
EOM	: External Ocular Movement.
EORTC	: European Organisation for Research and Treatment of Cancer.
Eos.	: Eosinophils
E/P	: Eicosapentaenoic Acid. (Ref. a dietary requirement).
EP	: Electrophysiology or Electrophysiological.

EPA   : Eicosapentaenoic Acid.
EPAs   : Extra Programmed Activities.
EPACT   : Electronic Prescribing Analysis and Cost.
EPAP   : Expiratory Positive Airway Pressure.
EPASS   : Educational Providers Accreditation Scheme. (Ref. used in Scotland).
EPB   : Epidural Blood Patch.
EPC   : Electronic Product Code.
               Epilepsia Partialis Continua.
EPEC   : Entero-Pathogenic Escherichia. Coli.
EPIC   : Evidence-based Practice in Infection Control.
EPLS   : European Paediatric Life Support.
EPMAR   : Erythropoietin (or Recombinant Human Erythropoieten).
EPO   : Erythropoietin.
EPOA   : Enduring Power of Attorney.
EPOS   : European Perspective Osteoporosis Study.
EPP   : Evaluation of Professional Practices.
               Expert Patient Programme.
EPQ   : Eysenk Personality Questionnaire.
EPR   : Electronic Patient Record.
EPS   : Electronic Prescribing (or Prescription) Service.
               Electrophysiological Study.
               Extrapyramidal Side effects. (Ref. with Anti-psychotic agents).
EPSEs   : Extra-Pyramidal Side Effects.
EPSP   : Excitatory Post-synaptic Potential.
EPU   : Early Pregnancy Unit.

EQUATOR   : Enhencing the Quality and Transparency of Health Research.

ER   : Emergency Regimen.
               Endoplasmic Reticulum.
               Oestrogen Receptor.
ERA   : European Renal Association.
ERC   : Endoscopic Retrograde Cholangiography.
ERCP   : Endoscopic Retrograde Cholangio-pancreatography.

ERG	: Electroretinogram.
ERK2	: Extra-Cellular Signal-Regulated Kinase 2.
ERLS	: Emergency Reference Levels.
ERPC	: Evacuation of Retained Products of Conception.
ERPOC	: Evacuation of Retained Products of Conception.
ERPF	: Effective Renal Plasma Flow.
ERS	: European Respiratory Society.
ERT	: Oestrogen Replacement Therapy.
ERV	: Expiratory Reserve Volume.
ES	: Endoscopic Sphincterotomy.
	Enema Saponis.
ESA	: End-Systolic Area.
	Erythropoiesis Stimulating Agents.
ESBL	: Extended Spectrum Beta-Lactamase.
ESC	: European Society of Cardiology.
ESF	: Established Renal Failure.
ESI	: Entire Soma Isolation (method). (Ref. a neuron excitability study).
ESICM	: European Society of Intensive Care Medicine.
ESM	: Ejection Systolic Murmur.
ESN	: Educationally Subnormal.
ESPEN	: European Society of Parenteral and Enteral Nutrition.
ESR	: Electronic Staff Record.
	European Society of Anaesthesiologists.
	Erythrocyte Sedimentation Rate.(Ref. blood test in inflammatory disorders).
ESRC	: Economic and Social Research Council.
ESRD	: End-Stage Renal Disease .
ESRF	: End Stage Renal Failure.
ESS	: Endoscopic Sinus Surgery.
	Epworth Sleepness Scale.
ESSQ	: Edinburgh Surgical Sciences Qualification.
EST	: Exercise Stress Test.
ESWL	: Extra-corporeal Shock Wave Lithotripsy.
ESWT	: Extracorporeal Shock Wave Therapy.
ET	: Embryo Transfer.

	End Tidal.
	Endotracheal (Tube).
	Essential Thrombocythemia.
	Essential Tremor.
ETA	: European Thyroid Association.
ETAC	: Electrothermally Assisted Capsulorrhaphy.
ETAG	: End Tidal Anaesthetic Gas.(Ref. in Awareness and depth of Anaesthesia).
ETCO₂	: End-Tidal Carbon Dioxide.
ETD	: Eustachian Tube Dysfunction.
ETEC	: Entero-Toxingenic Escherichia. Coli.
ETI	: Endo-Tracheal Intubation.
ETLA	: Endonasal Topical Local Anaesthesia.
ETOH	: Ethanol (or Alcohol).
ETOH-W/D	: Alcohol Withdrawal.
ETP	: Electronic Transfer of Prescriptions.
ETT	: Endo-Tracheal Tube.
	Examination in Theatre.
	Exercise Tolerance Test(ing).
ETU	: Epidural Top Up.
ETV	: End-Tidal Volume.
EUA	: Examination Under Anaesthesia.
EULAR	: European League Against Rheumatism.
EUM	: Examination under the Microscope. (Usually of the Ears).
EUROCAT	: European Register of Congenital Anomalies.
EUS	: Endoscopic Ultrasonography.
	Epiaortic Ultrasound Scanning.
	Examination Under Sedation.
EV	: Expired Volume.
	Electrical Velocimetry.
EVA	: Enlarged Vestibular Aqueduct Syndrome.
EVARs	: Endo-Vascular Aortic Aneurysm Repairs.
EVD	: External Ventricular Drainage. (Ref. Intracranial pressure reduction).

	Extra-Ventricular Drain. (Ref. used in reducing intracranial pressure).
EVE	: Epidural Volume Extension. (Ref. following Epidural administration).
EVLW	: Extra-Vascular Lung Water (Content).
EVOH	: Ethylene Vinylalcohol Copolymer. (Ref. contrast used in Embolysis).
EVLP	: Ex-Vivo Lung Perfusion.
EVS	: Endoscopic Variceal Sclerotherapy.
EWMA	: European Wound Management Association.
EWS	: Early Warning Scoring (system.)
EWTD	: European Working Time Directive.
EXIT	: Ex-Utero Intrapartum Treatment.
EXT	: Extubation. (Ref. in Anaesthesia).
Ez	: Eczema.
F	: Fahrenheit.
	Father.
	Female.
	Fever.
	Fluorine.
FA	: Fatty Acid.
	Femoral Artery.
	Fibrosing Alveolitis.
	Foetal Anomaly.
Fab	: Fragment antigen binding.
FAB	: French-American-British. (Ref. classification for Acute Leukaemias).
FABP	: Flat Anterior Bite Plane.
FABQ	: Fear Avoidance Beliefs Questionnaire.
FAC	: Fractional Area Change. (Ref. assessment of systolic Heart function).
FACH	: Forceps to After-coming Head.
FACS	: Fluorescence-Activated Cell Sorting or Sorter. (Ref. Apoptosis analysis).

FACTT	: Fluid and Catheter Treatment Trial.
FAD	: Familial Alzheimer`s Disease.
	Flavin Adenine Dinucleotide.
FADL	: Functional Activities of Daily Living.
FAED	: Food Avoidance Emotional Disorder.
FAM	: Fertility Awareness Method.
FAMM	: Familial Atypical Multiple Melanoma.
FAO	: Food and Agriculture Organisation (of the **UN**).
FAP	: Familial Adenomatous Polyposis.
FAQ	: Food Amount Questionnaire.
	Frequently Asked Questions.
FAQs	: Frequently Asked Questions.
FAS	: Foetal Alcohol Syndrome.
	Foreign Accent Syndrome.
FASA	: Federated Ambulatory Surgery Association. (USA).
FAST	: Focused Assessment with Sonography in Trauma.
	Foetal Acoustic Stimulation Test.
FB	: Foreign Body.
FBC	: Full Blood Count.
FBDG	: Food-based Dietary Guidelines.
FBF	: Forearm Blood Flow.
FBP	: Foetal Biophysical Profile.
FBS	: Fasting Blood Sugar.
	Foetal Blood Sample.
Fc	: Fragment crystallisable.
FC	: Febrile Convulsion.
FC (f/c)	: Film-coated.
FCE	: Finished Consultant Episode.
FCNS	: Foundation Course in Natural Sciences.
F-COPES	: Family Crisis-Oriented Personal Evaluation Scales.
FCPs	: First Contract Practitioners.
FCR	: Flexor Carpi Radialis.
FCU	: Flexor Carpi Ulnaris.
FDA	: Food and Drug Authority. (USA).

FDCA	: Food and Drug Cosmetic Act. (USA).
FDE	: Fixed Drug Eruption.
FDFG	: Free-Dermal Fat Graft.
FDG	: Fluoro-2-deoxy-D-Glucose.
FDG (18-FDG)	:18-Fluorodeoxyglucose. (Ref. used in Radiology).
FDP	: Flexor Digitorum Profundus.
FDPs	: Fibrin (or Fibrinogen) Degradation Products.
FDSRCS	: Fellow of Dental Surgery, Royal College of Surgeons.
Fe	: Ferric/Ferrous (Iron).
FEI	: Faecal Elastase1.(Ref. Test for Pancreatic Exocrine Insufficiency: **PEI**).
FEIBA	: Factor Eight (VIII) Inhibitor Bypassing Activity.
FEMG	: Facial Electromyography.
Fen	: Fenestration.
FES	: Functional Electrical Stimulation.
FESC	: Framework for procuring External Support to Commissioners.
FESE	: Flexible Endoscopic Swallowing Examination.
FESS	: Functional Endoscopic Sinus Surgery.
FET	: Forced Expiratory Technique.
FEV	: Forced Expired Volume.
FEV-1	: Forced Expiratory Volume in one second.
FFA	: Fellow of the Faculty of Anaesthetists. Free Fatty Acids.
FFB	: Femoro-Femoral Bypass.
FFLM	: Faculty of Forensic and Legal Medicine.
FFM	: Fat-Free Mass.
FFP	: Fresh Frozen Plasma.
FFQ	: Food Frequence Questionnaire.
FFR	: Fractional Flow Reserve.
FFS	: Fee-for Service. (USA).
FFTS	: Foeto-Foetal Transfusion Sequence.
FGF	: Fibroblast Growth Factor.

Fresh Gas Flow.(Ref. Anaesthetic Gas mixture administered to a patient).

FGM : Female Genital Mutilation.

FH : Family History.
Familial Hypercholestrolaemia.
Foetal Heart.

FHH : Familial Hypocalciuric Hypercalcaemia.
Foetal Heart Heard.

FHNH : Foetal Heart Not Heard.

FHO : Foundation House Officer.

FHR : Foetal Heart Rate.

FHS : Family Health Services.

FHSA : Family Health Services Authority.

FI : Fibrinogen.
Faecal Incontinence.

FiAA : (Inspired) Fraction of Anaesthetic Agent.

Fib : Fibrositis
Fibula.

FIC : Fascia Iliaca Compartment.

FICB : Fascia Iliaca Compartment Block.(Ref. nerve block administration).

FIGO : Federation (International) of Gynaecologists and Obstetricians.

F I I : Fabricated Induced Illness. (Ref. Munchausen Syndrome).

FiO₂ : Fraction of Inspired Oxygen.

FIND : Foundation for Innovative New Diagnosis.

FISH : Fluorescence in situ Hybridization.

FITC : Fluorescent Molecular Fluorescein Isothiocynate.

FIV : Feline Immunodeficiency Virus.

fL : Fentolitre.

FL : Femur Length; (of Foetus).
: Fluid Load.

FLAIR : Fluid Attenuation Inversion Recovery (Scans).

FLACC : Faces, Legs Activity Cry Consolability (Scale).

FLD : Frontal Lobe Degeneration.

FLG	: Filaggrin Gene.
FLS	: Fibreoptic-assisted Laryngoscopy.
FM	: Face Mask.
	Fat Mass.
fm	: Fiat mistura. (Ref. Latin for; "make a mixture").
F: M	: Female: Male (Ratio.)
FMEA	: Failure Mode and Effect Analysis (Tool).
FMF	: Familial Mediterranean Fever.(Ref. due to mutations of Pyrin gene leading to painful inflammatory process in abdomen, joints etc).
	Foetal Movement Felt.
FMN	: Flavin Mono-nucleotide.
FMRI (f.MRI)	: Functional Magnetic Resonance Imaging.
FMV	: Facemask Ventilation.
FN	: Facial Nerve.
FNA	: Fine Needle Aspirate (or Aspiration).
FNAC	: Fine Needle Aspiration Cytology.
FND	: Functional Neck Dissection.
FNE	: Fear of Negative Evaluation.
FNHTR	: Febrile Non-Haemolytic Transfusion Reaction.
FNIF	: Florence Nightngale International Foundation.
FOB	: Faecal Occult Blood.
	Fibre-optic Bronchoscope.
FOBT	: Faecal Occult Blood Testing.
FOE	: Fractional Oxygen Extraction.
FOG	: Fast Oxidative-glycolitic (Fibres).
FOI	: Fibro-optic Intubation.
	Freedom of Information (Act 2000).
FOOSH	: Fallen On Outstretched (left) Hand.
FOP	: Fibrodysplasia Ossificans Progressiva.(Ref. muscle ossification genetic disease).
FOS	: Fructo-Oligosaccharides.
FOSIT	: Feeling of Something in the Throat.
FP	: Food Poisoning.

	Foundation Programme.
FP 10	: Form for Prescription.
FP (*a*-FP)	: Alpha-Foetal Protein.
FPA	: Family Planning Association.
FPAD	: Fractionated Plasma Separation Adsorption and Dialysis (System).
FPC	: Family Planning Clinic. Family Practitioner Committee.
FPCert	: Family Planning Certificate.
FPG	: Fasting Plasma Glucose.
FPH	: Faculty of Public Health.
FPHVS	: First Parent Health Visitor Scheme.
FPL	: Flexor Polysis Longus.
FPM	: Faculty of Pain Management. First Pass Metabolism.
FPOS	: First Person on the Scene.
FPR	: False-Positive Rate.
FPS	: First Pass Success.
FRAX	: Fracture-Risk Assessment (Tool.)
FRAXA	: Fragile X Syndrome.
FRAXE	: Fragile-Site Mental Retardation.
FRC	: Feedback Reduction Circuit. Functional Residual Capacity.
FRCA	: Fellow of the Royal College of Anaesthetists.
FRcn	: Fellow of the Royal College of Nursing.
FRCOG	: Fellow of the Royal College of Obstetrics and Gynaecology.
FRCP	: Fellow of the Royal College of Physicians.
FRCPsych.	: Fellow of the Royal College of Psychiatry.
FRCR	: Fellow of the Royal College of Radiology.
FRCS	: Fellow of the Royal College of Surgeons.
FROM (FroM)	: Full Range of Movement.
FRSH	: Fellow of the Royal Society of Health.
FRV	: Functional Residue Volume.
FS	: Fundal-Symphyseal (height).
f/s	: Fissure sealant.

FSA	: Food Standards Agency.
FSE	: Feline Spongioform Encephalopathy.
	Foetal Scalp Electrode.
FSGS	: Focal Segmental Glomerulosclerosis.
FSH	: Follicle Stimulating Hormone.
FSS	: Fear Survey Schedule.
FT	: Flow Time
	Formol Toxoid.
	Full Term. (Ref. in Obstetrics).
FTc	: Flow Time (corrected).
FT3 (f.T3)	: Free Tri-iodothyronine.
FT4 (f.T4)	: Free Thyroxine.
FTA	: Fluorescent Treponemal Antibody. (Ref. Serology test for Syphilis).
FTA-ABS	: Fluorescent Treponemal Antibody Absorption (Test).
FTBD	: Fit to be detained.
	Full Term Born Dead.
FTD	: Frontotemporal Dementia.
FTE	: Full-Time Equivalent. (Ref. Employee cost calculations; USA).
FTI	: Free Thyroxine Index.
FTND	: Full Term Normal Delivery.
FTP	: Fitness to Practice.
FTSG	: Full-Thickness Skin Graft.
FTSTA	: Fixed Term Specialist Training Appointment.
FTT	: Failure to Thrive
FTU	: Finger-tip Unit.
FU (5–FU)	: 5-Fluorouracil. (Ref. a chemotherapeutic agent).
FUO	: Fever of Unknown Origin.
FV	: Femoral Vein.
FVC	: Forced Vital Capacity.
FVL	: Factor V Leiden. (Ref. Genetic mutant associated with Thrombophilia).
FVR	: Forearm Vascular Resistance.

FW : Forced Whisper.

Fx : Fracture.

FY 1 : Foundation Year 1 (Trainee).

g. : Gram.
G : Gauge.
G & A : Gas and Air.
GA : General Anaesthesia.
Granuloma Annulare.
GABA : Gamma Amino Butyric Acid.
GABEB : Generalised Atrophic Begnin Epidermolysis Bullosa.
GABHS : Group A *B*-Haemolytic Streptococcus.
GAD : Generalised Anxiety Disorder.
Glutamic Acid Decarboxylase.
GAF : Global Assessment of Functioning (Scale).
GAG : Glycosaminoglycan.
GAIN : Global Alliance for Improved Nutrition.
GAIT : Glucosamine/Chondroitin Arthritis Intervention Trial.
GALT : Gut-Associated Lymphoid Tissue.
GAMA : Gamma Amino-Buteric Acid.
GANFYD : Get A Note From Your Doctor.
GAP : Gravity Assisted Positioning.
GAPDH : Glyceradehyde-3-phosphate.
GARS : Gait Abnormality Rating Scale.
GAS : General Adaptation Syndrome.
Glasgow Aneurysm Score.(Ref. post-op mortality
prediction in Triple **A**).
Group A Streptococci.
GAT(Sanford): Sanford Guide to Antimicrobial Therapy.
GAVI : Global Alliance for Vaccines and Immunisation.

GB : Gall-bladder.
GBHP : Glomerular Blood Hydrostatic Pressure.
GBM : Glomerular Basement Membrane.
GBR : Guided Bone Regeneration.
GBS : Group B Streptococcus.

Guillian-Barre Syndrome.
GBSI : Group B Streptococcal Infection.

GC : General Condition.
Gonococcus.
GCA : Giant Cell Arthritis.
GCC : General Chiropractic Council.
GCFT : Gonococcal Complement Fixation Test.
GCK : Glucokinase.
GCP : Good Clinical Practice.
GCRP : Good Clinical Research Practice.
GCS : Glasgow Coma Score.
G-CSF : Granulocyte Colony-Stimulating Factor. (Ref. used in Traumatic Brain Injury to improve immune function).

GCT : Germ Cell Tumour.
Giant Cell Tumour.
GDA : Guideline Daily Amount.
GDC : Guglielmi Detachable Coil.(Ref. used to occlude cerebral aneurysms).
General Dental Council.
GDG : Guideline Development Group. (U.K).
GDM : Gestational Diabetes Mellitus.
GDP : General Dental Practitioner.
Guanosine Diphosphate.
GDS : Genatric Depression Scale.
General Dental Services.
Geriatric Depression Scale.

GEB : Gum Elastic Bougie.

GER : Gastroesophageal Reflux.
GERD : Gastroesophageal Reflux Disease.
GERI : Geriatrics.

GET : Graded Exercise Therapy.

GF : Glomerular Filtration.

Gluten-Free.
Granuloma Faciale.
GFAP : Glial Fibrillary Acidic Protein.(Ref. used in Immunocytochemistry).
GFR : Glomerular Filtration Rate.

GGT : Gluconyl-Glycyl Transaminase.
GGTP : Gamma-glutamyl Transpeptidase.

GH : Growth Hormone.
Gynaecological History.
GHb : Glycerated Haemoglobin.
GHB : Gamma-hydroxybutyrate.
Gammahydroxybutyric Acid.
GHD : Growth Hormone Deficiency.
GvHD : Graft versus Host Disease.
GHIH : Growth Hormone Inhibiting Hormone.
GHIS : Growth Hormone Insensitivity Syndrome.
GHQ : General Health Questionnaire.
GHRH (GRH) : Growth Hormone-Releasing Hormone.
GHRIH : Growth Hormone Release-Inhibiting Hormone.
GHS : General Household Survey.

GI : Gastro-Intestinal.
Glycaemic Index.
GIFT : Gamete Intrafallopian Transfer.
GIK : Glucose-Insulin-Potassium (Therapy).
GIM : General Internal Medicine.
GIP : Gastric Inhibitory Polypeptide.
GIS : Gastrointestinal System.
GIST : Gastro-Intestinal Stomal Cell Tumour.
GIT : Gastro-Intestinal Tract.

GKI : Glucose, Potassium, Insulin (infusion).

GL : Glycaemic Load.
glc : Glucose.
gln : Glutamine.

GLP-1	: Glucagon-like Peptide Type 1.
gm	: Gram.
GM	: Gluteus Medius (muscle). (USA).
GMC	: General Medical Council.
GMFA	: Gay Men Fighting **AIDS.**
GMO	: Genetically Modified Organism.
GMP	: Good Medical Practice.
	Guanosine Monophosphate.
	Guide to good Manufacturing Practice.
GMS	: General Medical Services.
GMSC	: General Medical Services Committee.
GMSPS	: Glasgow Meningococcal Septicaemia Prognostic Score.
GN	: Glomerulonephritis.
GNB	: Gram-Negative Bacteria.
GnRH	: Gonadotrophin-Releasing Hormone.
GO	: Global Oximetry. (Ref. a project by **WHO** in Developing Countries under the banner "Safe Surgery Saves Lives").
GOA	: Generalised Osteo-Arthritis.
GOR	: Gastro-Oesophageal Reflux.
GORD	: Gastro-Oesophageal Reflux Disease.
GOS	: Glasgow Outcome Scale.
GP	: General Practitioner.
	Glycoprotein.
	Gutta-Percha.
GPx	: Glutathione Peroxide.
GPAQ	: General Practice Assessment Questionnaire.
GPC	: Gastric Parietal Cell.
	General Physical Condition.
	General Practitioners Committee.
G6PD	: Glucose-6-Phosphatase Deficiency.
	Glucose 6-Phosphate Dehydrogenase.
GPE	: Global Perceived Effect. (Ref. extremes of pain levels).
GPEP	: Graduate and Professional Entry Programme.
GPFC	: General Practice Finance Corporation.

GPHIN : Global Public Health Intelligence Network.
GPI : General Paralysis of the Insane.
GPN : General Practice Nurse.
GPP : Good Publication Practice.
GPRD : General Practice Research Database.
GPSI (GPwSI): General Practitioner with Special Interest.
GPs4Y : General Practitioners for Young People.

GRADE : Grading of Recommendations Assessment,
Development and Evaluation.
(Ref. Clinical recommendations versus Resource use).
GRCA : Glasgow Register of Congenital Abnormalities.
GRID : Gay Related Immune Deficiency.
GRV : Gastric Residual Volume.

GS : Glidescope. (Ref. a Video Laryngoscope used
in Anaesthesia).
G & S : Group and Save (Serum for Blood Transfusion).
GSCC : General Social Care Council.
GSD : Gallstone Disease.
Glycogen Storage Disease.
GSI : Genuine Stress Incontinence.
GSK : GlaxoSmith Kline. (Ref. the International
Pharmaceutical Company).
GSL : General Sales List. (Ref. of Medical Products). (USA).
GSM : Global System Mobile. (Ref. the Transmission of
Telemedicine Data).

GT : Glucose Tolerance Test.
GTA : Gynaecology Teaching Assistants. (Ref. the women
used for Vaginal Examinations in Gynaecology).
GTAC : Gene Therapy Advisory Committee.
GTD : Gestational Trophoblastic Disease.
GTN : Glycyl Trinitrate.
GTO : Golgi Tendon Organ. (Ref. sensory organ in muscle
fibres).
GTP : Gestational Thrombocytopenia of Pregnancy.
Guanosine Triphosphate.

GTR	: Guided Tissue Regeneration.
GTT	: Gestational Trophoblastic Tumour.
	Glucose Tolerance Test.
GU	: Gastric Ulcer.
	Genito-Urinary.
GUCH	: Grown-Up Congenital Heart Disease.
GUD	: Genital Ulcer Disease.
GUM	: Genito-Urinary Medicine.
GUS	: Genito-Urinary System.
GUSTO	: Global Utilisation of Streptokinase and **t-PA** for occluded Coronary Arteries.
GUT	: Genital Urinary Tract.
GVA	: General Visceral Afferent (fibers). (USA).
GVE	: General Visceral Efferent (fibers). (USA).
GVHD	: Graft versus Host Disease.
GWA	: Genome-Wide Association (Studies). (Ref. a study of Genetic Diseases).
GWC	: General Whitley Council.
GYN(Gynae.)	: Gynaecology.
h **(hr)**	: Hour.
H	: Hospital.
	Hydrogen.
H2	: Histamine 2–receptor Antagonist.
HA	: Haemagglutination.
	Headache.
	Health Authority.
	Hyaluronic Acid.
HAA	: Hepatitis Associated Antigen.
HAART	: Highly Active Anti-retroviral Therapy.
	Highly Articulate Angry Reaction to Teaching.
HABP	: Hyaluronic Acid-Binding Protein.
HACCP	: Hazard Analysis Critical Control Points.
HACE	: High Altitude Cerebral Oedema.

HACEK : Haemophilus, Acintobacillus, Cardiobacterium, Ekenella and Kingella.

HACT : Hemochron Activated Clotting Time.

HAD : Health Development Agency.
Hospital Anxiety and Depression Questionnaire.

HADS : Hospital Anxiety and Stress Scale.

HAE : Heriditary Angioedema.

HAIs : Hospital Acquired Infections.

HAIgM : Hepatitis A Ig M.

HALE : Health Adjustment Life Expectancy.

HAMAT : Hazardous Materials.

HAPE : High Altitude Pulmonary Oedema. (Oedema is UK; Eodema is USA)

HAPO : High Altitude Pulmonary Oedema. (Oedema is UK; Eodema is USA).
Hyperglycaemia and Adverse Pregnancy Outcome. (see under **IHAPO**).

HAQ : Health Assessment Questionnaire.

HAS : Hepatic Artery Stenosis.
Human Albumin Solution.
Hamilton Anxiety Scale.

HAT : Hepatic Artery Thrombosis.
Home Automated Trial. (Ref. trial with External Defibrillator).

HATI : Human Anti-Tetanus Immunoglobulin.

HATS : Hunter Area Toxicology Service.(Ref. in Serotonergic Drug Overdose).

HAV : Hepatitis A Virus.

HB : Health Board.
Hepatitis B.

Hb : Haemoglobin.

HbA : Adult Haemoglobin.

HbA1c : (Glycosylated) Haemoglobin. (Ref. for type 2 Diabetes Test).

HbAS : Sickle Cell Trait (Haemoglobin).

Hb-b : Haemoglobin concentration.

HBc : Hepatitis B core.

HBD	: Heart Beating Donor.
	Hydroxy-butyrate Dehydrogenase.
HBeAg	: Hepatitis B e Antigen (or Hepatitis B Core Antigen).
HbF	: Foetal Haemoglobin.
HBG	: Health Benefit Group.
HBGM	: Home Blood Glucose Monitoring.
HBI	: Heart Beat to Beat Interval.
HBID	: Hereditary Begnin Intraepithelial Dyskeratosis.
HBIg	: Hepatitis B Immuno-globulin.
HBL	: Hepatoblastoma.
HBO	: Hyperbaric Oxygen.
HBOCs	: Haemoglobin-Based Oxygen Carriers.
HBOT	: Hyperbaric Oxygen Therapy.
HBsAg	: Hepatitis B surface Antigen.
HBS	: Hypnotic-Based Sedation.
HbS	: Hepatitis B Surface.
	Sickle Cell Haemoglobin.
HbS-Bthal.	: Sickle Cell Beta Thalassaemia.
HbSC	: Sickle Cell Haemoglobin C (Disease).
HbSS	: Sickle Cell Anaemia.
HBV	: Hepatitis B Virus.
	High Biological Value.
HC	: Head Circumference (of a Foetus).
HCA	: Health Care Assistant.
HCAI	: Health Care Associated Infections.
HCC	: Healthcare Commission.
	Hepatocellular Cancer (or Carcinoma).
HCG (h.CG)	: Human Chorionic Gonadotrophin.
HCHS	: Hospital and Community Health Services.
HCl	: Hydrochloride (or Hydrochloric Acid).
HCM	: Hypertrophic Cardiomyopathy.
HCMP (HMPC)	: Herbal Medicinal Products Committee. (USA).
HCO₃	: Bicarbonate.
HCP	: Health Care Professionals.
	Health Care Projects.
	Health Care Providers.
HCQ	: Hydroxychloroquine.

H`CRIT (Hct) : Haematocrit.
HCSS　　　: Hypersensitive Carotid Sinus Syndrome.
HCTZ　　　: Hydrochlorothiazide.
HCV　　　: Hepatitis C Virus.
HCW　　　: Health Care Workers.

HD　　　　: Haemodialysis.
　　　　　　　Hirschsprung`s Disease.
　　　　　　　Hodgkin`s Disease.
　　　　　　　Huntington`s Disease (Chorea).
HDBB　　　: Horizontal Diagonal Bands of Broca.
HdF　　　 : Head of Femur.
HDL　　　 : High-Density Lipoprotein (or Lipids).
HDL-C　　 : High-Density Lipoprotein Cholesterol.
HDN　　　 : Haemolytic Disease of the Newborn.
HDU　　　 : High Dependence Unit.
HDV　　　 : Hepatitis Delta Virus.

HE　　　　: Heriditary Elliptocytosis.
HEFCE　　 : Higher Education Funding Council for England.
HELLP　　 : Haemolysis Elevated Liver Enzymes and Low
　　　　　　　Platelets Count (Syndrome).
　　　　　　　Haemolytic Anaemia-related Liver Enzymes-Low
　　　　　　　Platelet (Count).
HEMS　　　: Helicopter Emergency Medical Service.
Hep B　　 : Hepatitis B.
HES　　　 : Hydroxyethyl Starch.
　　　　　　　Hospital Episode Statistics.
HEV　　　 : Hepatitis E Virus.

HF　　　　: Haemofiltration.
　　　　　　　Hageman Factor.
HFEA　　　: Human Fertilisation and Embryology Authority.
HFO　　　 : High Frequency Oscillation.
HFOV　　　: High Frequency Oscillatory Ventilation.
HFS　　　 : Health Facilities in Scotland.

Hg　　　　: Mercury.

H3G	: Hydromorphone-3-Glucuronide.
HGC	: Human Genetic Commission.
HGF	: Haematopoietic Factor.
hGH	: Human Growth Hormone.
HGP	: Human Genome Project.
HGV	: Hepatitis G Virus.

HH	: Hiatus Hernia.
	Hypogonadotrophic Hypogonadism.
H@H	: Hospital at Home.
HHC	: Helen Hanlyn Centre. (Ref. Design centre for patients safety; see **DPS**).
HHNK	: Hyperglycaemic Hyperosmolar Non-Ketotic.
HHS	: Health and Human Services. (USA).
	Hyperosmolar Hyperglycaemic Syndrome.
HHT	: Heriditary Haemorrhagic Telangiectasia.
HHV	: Human Herpes Virus.

HI	: Haemagglutination Inhibition.
	Head Injury.
HIA	: Health Impact Assessment.
	Health Improvement Assessment.
HIAA	: Hydroxyindoleacetic Acid.

HIB (Hib)	: Haemophilus influenzae type B (Vaccine).
HICPAC	: Hospital Infection Control Practices Advisory Committee.
HIDA	: Hepato-Immunodiacetic Acid.
HIDS	: Hyper-IgD Syndrome.(Ref. Autosomal recessive disorder; see **FMF**).
HIE	: Hypoxic Ischaemic Encephalopath.
HIECs	: Health Innovation and Education Clusters. (Ref. Biomedical research into **NHS** practice for patients benefit).
HIES	: Hyper IgE Syndrome.(Ref. Primary Immunodeficiency Disease).
HIF	: Hypoxia Induced Factor.
HIMP	: Health Improvement and Modernisation Plan.

HImpP   : Health Improvement Programme.
HIPAA   : Health Insurance Portability and Accountability. (USA).
HIPEC   : Hyperthermic Intraperitoneal Chemotherapy.
                     (Ref. peritoneal myesothelioma Chemotharapy).
HIS   : Health Information System.
HIT   : Heparin-Induced Thrombocytopenia.
HIV   : Human Immunodeficiency Virus. (Ref. Previously
                     known as **HTLV-3**).
HIW   : Health Inspectorate (of) Wales.

HL   : Hairy Leukoplakia.
HLA   : Histocompatibility Antigen.
                     Human Leucocytes Antigen.
HLH   : Haemophagocytic Lymphohistiocytosis.
HLHS   : Hypoplastic Left Heart Syndrome.
HLT   : Heart Lung Transplant.

HM   : Head Movements.
HMC   : Hospital Management Committee.
HMD   : Hyaline Membrane Disease.
HME   : Heat and Moisture Exchanger.

HMEFs   : Humidification and Heat Exchanger Filters.
                     Hygrobaby Heat and Moisture Exchanger Filters.
HMG(Hmg)   : Human Menopausal Gonadotrophin.
HMG-CoA   : 3-Hydroxy-3 Methyl-glutaryl Co-Enzyme A.
HMMA   : Hydroxymethylmandelic Acid (or 4-Hydroxy-3-
                     Methoxymandelic Acid).
HMOs   : Health Maintenance Organizations. (USA).
HMWK   : High Molecular Weight Kininogen. (Ref. in blood
                     clot formation.)

HNA   : Health Needs Assessment.
                     Heparin Neutralising Activity.
HNCM   : Hypertrophic Non-Obstructive Cardiomyopathy.
HND   : Haemolytic Disease of the Newborne.
HNIG   : Human Normal Immunoglobulin.
HNP   : Herniated Nucleus Pulposus.

HNPCC	: Heriditary Non-polyposis Colon/Colorectal Cancer (syndrome.)
HNPU	: Has Not Passed Urine.

H₂O	: Water.
HO	: House Officer.
HO-I	: Haemo-Oxygenase 1.
h/o	: History of.
HOAC 11	: Hypothesis-Oriented Algorithm for Clinicians 11.
HOCM	: Hypertrophic Obstructive Cardiomyopathy.
HoF (H of F)	: Height of Fundus (i.e Fundal Height in Obstetrics).
HOMA	: Homeostasis Model Assessment.
HOMA-IR	: Homeostasis Model Assessment of Insulin Resistance.
HONK (HONC)	: Hyper-Osmolar Non-Ketotic Coma.
HoNOS	: Health of the Nation Outcomes Scales.
HOP	: High Oxygen Pressure.
HOT	: Hypertensive Optimal Treatment.
HOTCAFE	: How to Treat Atrial Fibrillation.
HOWIS	: Health of Wales.

HP	: Hydrogen Peroxide.
HPA	: Health Protection Agency.
	Human Platelet Antigen.
	Hypothalamo-Pituitary Adrenal Axis.
HPC	: Health Professions Council.
	History of Present Complaint (or Condition).
HPDT	: Heat Pain Detection Threshold.
HPE	: Holoprosencephaly.
HPF	: High-Power Field.
HPFH	: Heriditary Persistence of Foetal Haemoglobin.
HPL (hPL)	: Human Placental Lactogen.
HPLC	: High Performance Liquid Chromatography.
HPMA	: Healthcare People Management Association.
HPO	: Hypothalamopituitary-Ovarian (axis).
HPOA	: Hypertrophic Pulmonary Osteoarthropathy.
HPP	: Heriditary Pyropoikilocytosis.
	Hypokalaemic Periodic Paralysis.

HPS	: Hermansky-Pudlak Syndrome.(Ref. syndrome of; Oculocutaneous Albinism, a bleeding tendency plus Lipofuscinosis).
HPSS	: Health and Personal Social Services (of Northern Ireland).
HPT	: Hyperparathyroidsm. Hpothalamo-Pituitary-Throid (Axis).
HPV	: Human Papilloma Virus. Hypoxic Pulmonary Vasoconstriction.
HQIP	: Healthcare Quality Improvement Partnership.
HR	: Hazard Ratio. (Ref. in Statistical analysis). Heart Rate. Hold-Relax (Procedure in Orthopaedics).
HRA	: High Right Atrium.
HRB	: Health Reserve Board.
HRCT	: High-Resolution Computerised Tomography.
HRG	: Health Care Resource Groups.
HRQOL	: Health Related Quality of Life.
HRR	: Heart Rate Reserve.
HRT	: Hormone Replacement Therapy.
HRV	: Heart-Rate Variability.
HS	: Heriditary Spherocytosis.
HSA	: Hospital Savings Association. Human Serum Albumin.
HSC	: Health and Safety Commission. Health Service Circular. Health Select Committee.
HSCA	: Health and Social Care Authority (of Northern Ireland).
HSCB	: Health and Social Care Board.
HSCI	: Health Service Cost Index.
HSCT	: Haematopoietic Stem Cell Transplantation. (Ref. Primary Immunodeficiency Disease Treatment). Health and Social Care Trust. (Northern Ireland).
HSD	: Hydroxy-Steroid Dehydrogenase.
HSDU	: Hospital Sterilisation and Disinfection Unit.

HSE	: Health Safety Executive.
	Herpes Simplex Encephalitis.
HSG	: Hystero-Salpingogram.
HSM	: Hepatosplenomegaly.
HSP	: Henoch-Schonlein Purpura.
HSSB	: Health and Social Services Board (of Northern Ireland).
HSSC	: Health and Social Services Council (of Northern Ireland).
HST	: Higher Surgical Training.
HSV	: Herpes Simplex Virus.
HSVE	: Herpes Simplex Virus Encephalitis.
Ht	: Height.
HT (HTN)	: Hypertension.
HT (5-HT)	: 5–Hydroxytriptamine.
HTA	: Health Technology Assessment (Programme).
	Hierarchical Task Analysis
	Human Tissue Act.
	Human Tissue Authority.
HTIG	: Human Tetanus Immunoglobin.
HTLV-3	: Human T-Cell Lymphotrophic Viruses.(Now **HIV**).
	Human T-Cell Leukaemia Virus.
HTO	: High Tibial Osteotomy of the Knee.
HU	: Hounsfield Units. (Ref. attenuation value in **CT** terms).
HUS	: Haemolytic Ureamic Syndrome.
HV	: Health Vistor.
	Health Volunteer.
HVA	: Homo-Vanillic Acid.
HVCert	: Health Visitor Certificate.
HVHF	: High Volume Haemofiltration
HVLA	: High Velocity Low Amplitude (Thrust Technique).
HVLT	: High Velocity Thrust. (Ref. in the treatment of locked facet).
HVS	: High Vaginal Swab.
	Hyperventilation Syndrome.
HVT	: Health Visitor Teacher.

Hx	: Haemorrhage
	History.
Hycosy.	: Hystero-Salpingo Contrast Sonography.
HYMS	: Hull York Medical School.
Hz	: Hertz (Cycles per second).
I	: Increased.
	Iodine.
IA	: Intra-Arterial.
	Intra-Articular.
IA(i/at)	: Intra-articular (administration).
IAA	: Insulin Auto-Antibody.
IAAS	: International Association for Ambulatory Surgery.
IABP	: Intra-Aortic Balloon Pump.
IAC	: Internal Auditory Canal.
IADL	: Instrumental Activities of Daily Living (Scale).
IADPSG	: International Association of Diabetis in Pregnancy Study Group.
IADs	: Internal Automated Defibrillators.(Ref. management of Cardiomyopathy).
IAN	: Inferior Alveolar Nerve.
IAP	: Intra-abdominal Pressure.
IAPP	: Islet Amyloid Polypeptide.
IAPT	: Improved Access to Psychological Therapies.
IARC	: International Agency for Research on Cancer.
IASP	: International Association for Study of Pain.
IBD	: Inflammatory Bowel Disease.
	Irritable Bowel Disease.
IBS	: Irritable Bowel Syndrome.
IBTICM	: Intercollegiate Board for Training in Intensive Care Medicine.
IBW	: Ideal Body Weight.
IC	: Intermittent Claudication.

	Interstitial Cystitis.
	Intracardiac.
ICA	: Internal Carotid Artey.
	Islet Cell Antibodies.
ICAM	: Intercellular Adhesion Molecules.(Ref. in atherosclerotic plaque formation).
ICAS	: Independent Complaints Advocacy Service.
ICBTICM	: Intercollegiate Board for Training in Intensive Care Medicine (Ref. see under **IBTICM**).
ICD	: Implantable Cardiac Defibrillator. Intercostal Drain. International Classification of Diseases.
ICDs	: Impulse Control Disorders. (Ref. e.g in Parkinson Disease: **PD**).
ICDH	: Isocitric Dehydrogenase.
ICDSC	: Intensive Care Delirium Screening Checklist.
ICE	: Incremental Clinical Examination. Intra-Cardiac Echo.
ICER	: Incremental Cost Effective Ratio. (Ref. a model in costing treatments).
ICF	: Intermediate Care Facility. Intra-Cellular Fluid.
ICG	: Impendance Cardiography.
ICH	: International Conference on Harmonising Pharmaceuticals for human use. Intra-cerebral Haemorrhage. Intra-Cranial Hypertension.
ICHC	: Independent Community and Health Concern.
ICIDH	: International Classification of Impairments, Disabilities, and Handicaps.
ICM	: Intensive Care Medicine. International Confederation of Midwives.
ICMA	: Intra-Cranial Myocotic Aneurysm.
ICMJE	: International Committee of Medical Journal Editors.
ICN	: Infection Control Nurse. International Council of Nurses.
ICNA	: Infection Control Nurses`s Association.

ICNARC   : Intensive Care National Audit and Research Centre.
ICP   : Integrated Care Pathways..
               Intercuspal Position.
               Intracranial Pressure.
ICPs   : Integrated Care Pathways.
ICRP   : International Commission on Radiological Protection.
ICRS   : Integrated Care Records Service.
ICS   : Intensive Care Society.
ICSDs   : International Classification of Sleep Disorders.
ICSH   : Interstitial Cell-Stimulating Hormone.
ICSI   : Intracytoplasmic Sperm Injection.
ICSRs   : Individual Case Safety Reports. (USA).
ICSS   : International Carotid Stenting Study.
ICT   : Infection Control Team.
               Information and Communication Technology.
               Inguinal Compression in Trendelenburg (position).
ICU   : Intensive Care Unit.

Id   : Intradermal.
ID   : Identification.
               Infectious Disease.
               Inferior Dental.
               Internal Diameter.
               Identification Document.
I&D   : Incision and Drainage.
IDA   : Iron Deficiency Anaemia.
IDB   : Inferior Dental Block.
IDD   : Iodine Deficiency Disorder.
IDDM   : Insulin Dependent Diabetes Mellitus.
IDL   : Intermediate-density Lipoproteins.
IDM   : Infant of Diabetic Mother.
IDNT   : Irbesartan Diabetic Neuropathy Trial.
IDPN   : Intradialytic Parenteral Nutrition.
IDS   : Intubation Difficulty Scale. (Ref. used in Anaesthetic
               practice).
               Inventory for Depressive Symptomatology.
IDUs   : Injection Drug Users.

IE	: Infective Endocarditis.
I: E	: Inspiratory time to Expiratory time Ratio.
IED	: Intubating Efficient Dosage.(Ref. Remifentanil use in General Anaesthesia).
IEF	: Isoelectric Focusing.
IEFSS	: Instrumental and Expressive Functions of Social Support.
IEIS	: Idiopathic Environmental Intolerance Syndrome. (Ref. previously **MCSS**).
IELTS	: International English Language Testing System.
IEM	: Inborn Error of Metabolism.
IEP	: Immunoelectrophoresis. Individual Education Plan.
IF	: Immunofluorescence. Intestinal Failure.
IFAPP	: International Federation of Associations of Pharmaceutical Physicians.
IFB	: Ilio-Femoral Bypass.
IFCC	: International Federation of Clinical Chemistry (and Laboratory Medicine).
IFG	: Impaired Fasting Glycaemia.
IFN-B	: Interferon-beta (or beta-Interferon.)
IFN-a	: Interferon-alpha.
IFT (m.IFT)	:(Modified) Isolated Forearm Technique.
IG	: Insulin Glargine.
Igs	: Immunoglobulins.
IgA	: Immunoglobulin A.
IGADS	: Investigator Global Assessment of Disease Status.
IgD	: Immunoglobulin D.
IgE	: Immunoglobulin E.
IgG	: Immunoglobulin G.
IgM	: Immunoglobulin M.
IGF-I	: Insulin-like Growth Factor 1
IGFs	: Insulin Growth Factors.
IGP	: Intra-Gastric Pressure.
IGRs	: Interferon Gamma Release Assays. (Ref. used in Tuberculosis Assay).

IGT   : Impaired Glucose Tolerance.
IGTT   : Impaired Glucose Tolerance Test.

IH   : Idiopathic (familial) Hirsutism.
                Inguinal Hernia.
IHA   : Independent Healthcare Association.
                Indirect Haemagglutination.
IHAPO : International Hyperglycaemia and Adverse Pregnancy
                Outcomes (Study).
IHAS   : Independent Healthcare Advisory Services.
IHCA   : In-Hospital Cardiac Arrest.
IHD   : Intermittent Haemodialysis.
                Ischaemic Heart Disease.
IHF   : International Hospitals Federation.
IHN   : Ilio-Hypogastric Nerve.
IHPS   : Idiopathic Hypertrophic Pyloric Stenosis.

IIA   : Internal Iliac Artery.
IIDB   : Industrial Injuries Disablement Benefit.
IIF   : Indirect Immunofluorescence.
IIN   : Ilio-Inguinal Nerve.
IIMs   : Idiopathic Inflammatory Myopathies.

IJD   : Inflammatory Joint Disease.
IJOA   : International Journal of Obstetric Anaesthesia.
IJV   : Internal Jugular Vein.

IL   : Interleukin.
                Intralesional.
ILA   : Individual Learning Account.
                Interventional Lung Assist.
ILAR   : International League of Associations for Rheumatology.
ILCOR : International Liaison Committee on Resuscitation.
ILD   : Interstitial Lung Disease.
ILE   : Intravenous Lipid Emulsion.
ILEA   : Intermittent Labour Epidural Analgesia.
ILP   : Inter-professional Learning in Practice.
ILS   : Immediate Life Support.

In-line Stabilisation.

IM	: Infectious Mononucleosis.
	Intermediate Metaboliser.
IM(i.m)	: Intra-muscular (Administration).
IMA	: Independent Midwives Association.
	Inferior Mesenteric Artery.
	Internal Mammary Artery.
IMAX	: Internal Maxillary (Artery).
IMB	: Intermenstrual Bleeding.
IMC	: Inter-Metacarpal (Joint).
IMCA	: Independent Mental Capacity Advocate.
IMD	: Inherited Metabolic Diseases.
IMEHD	: Implantable Middle Ear Hearing Device.
IMF	: Infra-Mammary Artery.
IMGs	: International Medical Graduates.
IMH	: Intramural Haematoma; (i.e in the Aorta).
IMIG	: Intra-muscular Immunoglobulin.
IMLs	: Intermediolateral Cell Columns (of the **CNS**). (USA).
IMPACT	: Ill Medical Patients Acute Care and Treatment.
	Improving Mood, Promoting Access to Collaborative Care Treatment.
Impr.	: Improved.
IMPs	: Investigational Medicinal Products. (USA).
IMRCS	: Intercollegiate Membership of the Royal College of Surgeons.
IMV	: Intermittent Mandatory Ventilation.
IN(i/n)	: Intra-Nasal.
IN	: Intubation. (Ref. in Anaesthesia).
Inc.	: Incisor (Tooth).
IND	: Investigational New Drug. (USA).
inf.	: Inferior.
INH	: Isoniazid (or by Inhalation).
INN (rINN)	: (Recommended) International Non-proprietary Name.
INO	: Inhaled Nitric Oxide.

Internuclear Ophthalmoplegia. (Ref. seen in damaged 6th Nerve with the adduction of the ipsilateral Eye).

INR : International Normalised Ratio.
Interventional Neuro-Radiology.

INRIG : Irish Nursing Research Interest Group.

INS : International Numbering System (for Food Additives).

INVEST : International Verapamil-Trandolapril Study.

in vitro : Latin for; "living in glass "; (A process or a reaction).

in vivo : Latin for;" in a living thing;."(A process taking place in a living organism).

IO : Intraosseous.

I & O : Intake and Output.

IOFBs : Intra-Ocular Foreign Bodies.

IOL : Induction of Labour.
Intra-ocular Lens.

IOP : Intra-Ocular Pressure.
Institute of Psychiatry.

IP : In-Patient.
Insurance Patient.
Interphalangeal.
Intra-Peritoneal.

IPA : Individual Practice Association. (USA).
Immunosupressive Acid Protein.

IPAP : Inspiratory Positive Airway Pressure.

IPC : Ischaemic Pre-Conditioning. (Ref. previously Transient Cardiac Ischaemia.)

IPCC : Inter-Professional Care Co-ordinator.

IPCU : Intensive Psychiatric Care Unit.

IPD : Idiopathic Parkinson`s Disease.
Intermittent Peritoneal Dialysis.

IPF : Idiopathic Pulmonary Fibrosis.

IPH : Idiopathic Pulmonary Haemosiderosis.

IPI : International Prognostic Index.

IPN : Infra-Patella Nerve.

IPP : Inter-pleural Pressure.

IPPB	: Intermittent Positive Pressure Breathing.
IPPV	: Intermittent Positive Pressure Ventilation.
IPSID	: Immuno-Proliferitive Small Intestine Disease.
IPSRT	: Interpersonal and Social Rhythms Therapy.
IPSS	: International Pilot Study of Schizophrenia.
IPT	: Interpersonal Therapy.
IPU	: Information Policy Unit (of the **DoH**).
IQ	: Intelligence Quotient.
IQR	: Interquartile Range. (Ref. in Statistics.)
IR	: Immediate Release. (Ref. formulation of a drug).
	International Radiology.
	Ischaemic Reperfusion.
IRA	: Infarct-related Artery (Coronary).
IRBs	: Institutional Review Boards. (USA).
IRBBB	: Incomplete Right Bundle Branch Block.
IRCT	: International Rehabilitation Council for Torture (Victims).
IRL	: Infrared Light.
IRMA	: Immunoradiometric Assay.
	Intra-retinal Microvascular Abnormalities.
IRRT	: Intermittent Renal Replacement Therapy.
IRT	: Immune Reactive Trypsinogen (or Trypsin).
IRV	: Inspiratory Reserve Volume.
IS	: Incentive Spirometry.
	Isotope Scanning.
ISA	: Intrinsic Sympathomimetic Activity.
ISAC	: Independent Scientific Advisory Committee.
ISAGA	: Immunosorbent Agglutination Assay.
ISAT	: International Sub-arachnoid Aneurysm Trial.
ISB	: Information Standards Board (of the **NHS**).
ISBPB	: Interscalene Brachial Plexus Block.
ISBT	: International Society for Blood Transfusion.
ISC	: Intermittent Self-Catheterisation.
ISCP	: Intercollegiate Surgical Curriculum Project.
ISDD	: Institute for the Study of Drug Dependence.

ISEIRE	: International Society for Exercise Intolerance Research and Education.
ISKDC	: International Study of Kidney Disease in Children.
ISMN	: Iso-sorbide Mono-nitrate.
ISMPP	: International Society for Medical Publication Professionals.
ISNs	: Integrated Service Networks. (USA).
ISO	: International Standards Organisation.
ISQ	: In Status Quo. (i.e no change).
ISRT	: International Spinal Resaerch Trust.
ISS	: Injury Severity Scale.
ISSHP	: International Society for the Study of Hypertension in Pregnancy.
ISSVD	: International Society for the Study of Vulval Diseases.
IST	: International Stroke Trial.
ISTCs	: Independent Sector Treatment Centres.
IT	: Iliotibial (Band in Orthopaedics.)
IT (i/t)	: Intra-Thecal; (a route of administration of drugs).
ITA	: Invasive Trophoblast Antigen.
ITBVI	: Intra-Thoracic Blood Volume Index.
ITc	: Intra-Thecal Catheter.
ITCP	: Idiopathic Thrombocytopenia Purpura.
ITFS	: Inducible Transcription Factors. (Ref. in the control of Gene expression).
ITGCN	: Intratubular Germ Cell Neoplasia.
ITm	: Intra-Thecal Morphine.
ITN	: Idiopathic Trigeminal Neuralgia.
ITP	: Idiopathic Thrombocytopenic Purpura. Immune Thrombocytopenia Purpura.
ITT	: Insulin Tolerance Test. Intention to Treat.
ITU	: Intensive Therapy (or Treatment) Unit.
ITx	: Intestinal Transplantation.
IU (i.u)	: International Unit. Intra-Uterine.
IUCD	: Intra-Uterine Contraceptive Device.

IUD	: Intra-Uterine Death.
	Intra-Uterine Device.
IUGR	: Intra-Uterine Growth Restriction.
	Intra-Uterine Growth Retardation.
IUI	: Intra-Uterine Insemination.
IUI + OI	: Intra-uterine Insemination plus Ovulation Induction.
IUP	: Intra-Uterine Pregnancy.
IUS	: Intra-Uterine System.
IUT	: Intrauterine Blood Transfusion.
IV	: Intervertebral (disc).
IV (i.v)	: Intravenous (Administration).
IVC	: Inferior Vena Cava.
IVCT	: In-vitro Contracture Testing.(Ref. in Malignant Hyperpyrexia testing).
IVD	: Instrumental Vaginal Delivery.
	Intervertebral Disk Disease.
IVDSA	: Intravenous Digital Subtraction Angiogram.
IVDUs	: Intravenous Drug Users.
IVF	: In vitro Fertilisation.
IVF-HIC	: In vitro Fertilisation with a High Insemination Concentration.
IVH	: Intra-ventricular Haemorrhage.(Ref. Cerebral Ventricular Haemorrhage).
IVHP	: Intravenous High Potency.
IVI	: Intravenous Infusion.
IVIG	: Intravenous Immunoglobin.
IV IgG	: Intravenous Immunoglobulin G.
IVM	: Intravital Microscopy.
IVNAA	: In-vivo Neutron Activation Analysis.
IVNC	: Isolated Left Ventricular Non-Compaction.
IVP	: Intravenous Pyelogram.
IVRA	: Intravenous Regional Analgesia.
IVRT	: Isovolumic Relaxation Time.
IVS	: Interventricular Septum.
IVT	: Intravenous Therapy.
	Intravenous Transfusion.
IVU	: Intravenous Urography (or Urogram).

IVUD : Intravenous Urodynamogram.
IVUS : Intravascular Ultrasound

IX (Ix) : Investigations.

IZS : Insulin Zinc Suspension.

JA : Joint Arthrodesis.
JACCOL : Jaundice, Anaemia, Clubbing, Cyanosis, Oedema, Lymphadenopathy.
JAM : Junctional Adhesion Molecule. (Ref. integral membrane proteins).
JAMA : Journal of the American Medical Association.

JCA : Juvenile Chronic Arthritis.
JCAHO : Joint Commission on Accreditation of Healthcare Organizations.(USA).
JCGP : Joint Council for General Practice.
JCV : John Cunningham Virus.
JCVI : Joint Committee on Vaccination and Immunisation. (USA).

JDC : Junior Doctors Committee.
JDM : Juvenile Dermatomyositis.

JFC : Joint Formulary Committee.

JGA : Juxtaglomerular Apparatus.
JGCs : Juxtaglomerular Cells.

JHCI : Joint Health Claims Initiative.

JIA : Juvenile Idiopathic Arthritis.

JLG : Joint Liaison Group.

JMF : Junior Members Forum.
JMML : Juvenile Myelomonocytic Leukaemia.

JNA : Juvenille Nasopharyngeal Angiofibroma.
JNKs (cJNKs) : C-Jun N-terminal Kinase.

JPS : Joint Position Sense.

JRA : Juvenile Rheumatoid Arthritis.
JRCPTB : Joint Royal Colleges of Physicians Training Board.

JSN : Joint Space Narrowing.

J tube : Jejunostomy tube.

JVP : Jugular Venous Pressure.

K + : Potassium.
KA : Keratoacanthoma.
Knee Aspiration.
k.cal : Kilocalories.
KCC : Kings College Criteria.(Ref. prognostic scoring system for Liver Transplant).
KCl : Potassium Chloride.
KCT : Kaolin Clotting Time.
KCCT : Kaolin Cephalin Clotting Time.
KCO : Diffusion Coefficient of Carbon Monoxide.(Ref. function test in Lung Surgery).

KD : Kawasaki Disease.
Ketogenic Diet.
KDOQI : Kidney Disease Outcomes Quality Initiative.
KDOQL : Kidney Disease Outcomes Quality of Life (Questionnaire).
kg : Kilogram.
KGF : Keratinocyte Growth Factor.
kJ : Kilojoule.

K-nail : Kuntscher nail.

Kod : Knocked out.
KOH : Potassium Hydroxide.
KONP : Keep Our National Health Service (**NHS**) Public.
kPa : Kilopascals.

KS : Kaposi`s Sarcoma.

KUB : Kidney, Ureter, Bladder. (Ref. for X-ray use).
kV : Kilovoltage.

K-wire : Kirschner wire.

L : Left.
Liter.
Liver.
Lumbar.
LA : Lactic Acidosis.
Latex Agglutination.
Left Atrium.
Local Anaesthetic.
Local Authority.
Lupus Anticoagulant.
LAAM : Levo-Alpha Acetylmethadol.
Lab. : Laboratory.
LACS : Lacunar Circulation Stroke.
LAD : Left Anterior Descending (Coronary) Artery.
Left Axis Deviation.
Leukocyte Adhesion Deficiency.
LADA : Latent Auto-Immune Diabetes in Adults.
LADY : Latent Auto-Immune Diabetes in Young.
LAGB : Laparoscopic Adjustable Gastric Band.
LAH : Left Anterior Hemiblock.
Left Atrial Hypertrophy.
LAK : Lymphokinase-activated Killer (Cell).
LAM : Lactation Amenorrhoea Method.
LAN : Lymphoadenopathy.
LAO : Left Anterior Oblique (Angiocardiogram).
LAP : Left Atrial Pressure.

	Leucine Aminopeptidase.
	Leukocyte Alkaline Phosphatase.
LARC	: Long-Acting Reversible (methods) Contraception.
LAS	: London Ambulance Service.
	Lymphadenopathy Syndrome.
LASIK	: Laser-Assisted in situ Keratomileusis.
LASS	: Local Authority Social Services.
LAT	: Lactate Anaerobic Threshold.
	Lidocaine, Adrenaline and Tetracaine.
	Locum Appointment for Training.
LATS	: Long-Acting Thyroid Stimulator.
LAUP	: Laser-Assisted Uvulopalatoplasty.

LB	: Live Birth.
	Liver Biopsy.
LBBB	: Left Bundle Branch Block.
LBM	: Lean Body Mass.
LBO	: Large Bowel Obstruction.
LBP	: Low (or Lower) Back Pain.
LBW	: Low Birth Weight.

LC	: Laparoscopic Cholecystectomy.
	Lymphocytic Colitis.
LCA	: Left Coronary Artery.
L-CAT	: Lecithin-Cholesterol Acetyl Transferase.
LCD	: Liquid Crystal Device (monitor).
	Liquid Crystal Display.
LCFA	: Long Chain Fatty Acids.
LCH	: Langaherans Cell Histiocytosis.
LCI	: Lung Clearance Index.(Ref. of ventilation in peripheral airway collapse).
LCL	: Lateral Collateral Ligament.
LCM	: Left Costal Margin.
LCMG	: Long Chain Monoglycerides.
LCP	: Liverpool Care Pathway.(Ref. care plan for terminally ill patients).
	Long Chain Polyunsaturated (Fatty Acids).
LCR	: Ligase Chain Reaction.

LCT	: Long Chain Triglycerides.
LCV	: Leukocytoclastic Vasculitis.
LCX	: Left Circumflex (Artery).
LD	: Lactate Dehydrogenase.
	Learning Disability.
LDA	: Left Dorsoanterior (Position of the Foetus).
LDCT	: Low Dose Spiral **CT.**
LDH	: Lactate (or Lactic) Dehydrogenase.
LDI	: Low-Dose Infusion. (e.g Epidural Infusion).
LDL	: Low-Density Lipoprotein (or Lipids.)
LDL-C	: Low-Density Lipoprotein-Cholesterol.
LDP	: Left Dorsoposterior Position (of the Foetus).
	Local Delivery Plan.
LDQ	: Leeds Dyspepsia Questionnaire.
LDTF	: Low Dose Tissue Factor.
LDV	: Lymphogranuloma Venereum.
LE	: Left Eye.
LE cells	: Lupus Erythematosus cells.
LEDs	: Light Emitting Diodes.
LEEP	: Loop Electrosurgical Excision Procedure.
LEHPZ	: Lower Oesophageal High Pressure Zone.
LEMS	: Lambert-Eaton Myasthenic Syndrome.
LEP	: Laparoscopic Extraperitoneal (approach).
LEPS	: Levitan F.P. Scope.(Ref. Intubating Laryngoscope used in Anaesthesia).
LER	: Loss of Eye Reflex.
LES	: Local Enhanced Service.
LESI	: Lumber Epidural Steroid Injection.
Lev.	: Levator (muscle).
LFA	: Left Fronto-Anterior (position of the Foetus).
LFH	: Lower Face Height.
LFP	: Left Fronto-Posterior (position of the Foetus).
LFTs	: Liver Function Tests
	Lung Function Tests.

LGA	: Large for Gestational Age.
LGIB	: Lower Gastro-intestinal Bleeding.
LGV	: Lymphogranuloma Venereum.
LH	: Luteinising Hormone.
LHA	: Local Health Authority.
LHB	: Local Health Board.
LHCC	: Local Healthcare Co-operative.
LHD	: Left Hemisphere(Brain) Damage.
LHG	: Local Health Group.
LHP	: Local Health Plan.
LHRH	: Luteinising Hormone Releasing Hormone.
LHSCG	: Local Health and Social Care Group (of Northern Ireland).
LHV	: Left Hepatic Vein.
LIA	: Local Infiltration Anaesthesia.
LICP	: Late Impair Cerebral Palsy.
LIF	: Left Iliac Fossa.
LIH	: Left Inguinal Hernia.
LIP	: Lymphoid Intestitial Pneumonitis (or Pneumonia).
LIPID	: Long-term Intervention with Pravastatin in Ischaemic Disease.
LIsegment	: Lumbar spine segment.
LIS	: Lung Injury Score.
LIT	: Lateral Infra-Clavicular Block. (Ref. in Anaesthetic practice).
LK	: Left Kidney.
LKM	: Liver, Kidney, Muscle. Liver, Kidney, Microsomal (Antibodies).
LL	: Lepromatous Leprosy.
LLETZ	: Large Loop Electrodiathermy Excision of the Transformation Zone.
LLL	: Left Lower Lobe.
LLQ	: Left Lower Quadrant (of the Abdomen).
LLS	: Lower Labial Segment.

LLZ	: Left Lower Zone.
LMA	: Laryngeal Mask Airway.
	Left Marginal Artery.
	Left Mento-Anterior (position of the Foetus).
LMC	: Local Medical Committee.
LMCA	: Left Main Coronary Artery.
LMN	: Lower Motor Neurone.
LMNLs	: Lower Motor Neurone Lesions.
LMP	: Last Menstrual Period.
	Left Mento-Posterior (position of the Foetus).
LMS	: Left Main Stem.
LMW	: Low Molecular Weight.
LMWH	: Low Molecular Weight Heparin.
LMZ	: Left Middle Zone.
LN	: Lymph Node.
LNC	: Local Negotiating Committee.
LND	: Lymph Node Dissection.
LNMP	: Last Normal Menstrual Period.
LOA	: Left Occipito-Anterior (position of the Foetus).
LOC	: Level of Consciousness.
	Loss of Consciousness.
LOCF	: Last Observation Carried Forward.
LOD	: Logistic Organ Dysfunction.
LODS	: Logistic Organ Dysfunction Score.
LOE	: Level of Evidence.
LOH	: Loss of Heterozygosity.
LOP	: Left Occipito-Posterior (position of the Foetus).
LORR	: Loss of Righting Reflex. (Ref. Propofol-induced Anaesthesia).
LOS	: Length of Stay.
	Loss of Sight.
	Lower Oesophageal Sphincter.
LOT	: Left Occipitotransverse.
LOX	: Lipoxygenases.

LP	: Lichen Planus.
	Lumbar Puncture.
LPA	: Lasting Power of Attorney.
	Latex Particle Agglutination.
LPC	: Left Pleural Cavity.
LPD	: Lymphoproliferative Disease.
LPH	: Left Posterior Hemiblock.
LPO	: Left Posterior Oblique. (Ref. an X-ray view).
LPR	: Lactate to Pyruvic Ratio(Ref. Biomaker of tissue ischaemia in Brain Injury).
LPS	: Lipopolysaccharide.
LPVS	: Lung Protective Ventilation Strategies.
LR	: Likelihood Ratio.
LRA	: Left Renal Artery.
LRD	: Living Related Donor.
LREC	: Local Research Ethics Committee.
LRNI	: Lower Reference Nutrient Intake.
LRT	: Likelihood Ratio Test.
LRTCs	: Lower Respiratory Tract Complications.
LRTI	: Lower Respiratory Tract Infection.
L: S	: Lecithin: Sphyngomyelin (Ratio).
LSC	: Legal Service Commission.
LSratio	: Lecithin-Sphingomyelin Ratio.
LSCS	: Lower Segment Caesarean Section.
LSD	: Lysergic Acid Diethylamide.
LSE	: Left Sternal Edge.
LSMT	: Life Sustaining Medical Treatment.
LSPs	: Local Service Providers.
LST	: Leishmanin Antigen Skin Test.
LTA	: Lipoteichoic Acid.
LTB	: Laryngotracheo-Bronchitis.
LTC	: Long-Term Care.
	Long-Term Condition.
LTFT	: Less Than Full Time Training.
LTM	: Long-term Memory.

LTOT : Long Term Oxygen Therapy.
LTP : Long Term Potentiation. (Ref. synaptic strength in pain pathways).
LTPP : Long Term Psychodynamic Psychotherapy.
LTRA : Leukotriene Receptor Antagonist.
LTS : Long Thermal Stimulation.

LUA : Left Upper Arm.
LUL : Left Upper Lobe (of the left Lung).
LUNA : Laparoscopic Uterine Nerve Ablation.
LUNSERS : Liverpool University Neuroleptic Side Effect Rating Scale.
LUQ : Left Upper Quadrant (of the Abdomen).
LUS : Laparoscopic Ultrasonography.
LUTO : Lower Urinary Tract Obstruction.
LUTS : Lower Urinary Tract Symptoms.
LUZ : Left Upper Zone.

LV : Left Ventricle.
Lumber Vertebra.
LVA : Left Visual Acuity.
LVAD : Left Ventricular Assist Device.
LVEDP : Left Ventricular End-diastolic Pressure.
LVEDV : Left Ventricular End-Diastolic Volume.
LVEF : Left Ventricular Ejection Fraction.
Left Ventricular End-diastolic Fraction
LVESV : Left Ventricular End-systolic Volume.
LVF : Left Ventricular Failure.
LVH : Left Ventricular Hypertrophy.
LVHT : Left Ventricular Hypertrabeculation.
LVIDD : Left Ventricular Internal Diastolic Dimension.
LVISD : Left Ventricular Internal Systolic Dimension.
LVIT : Left Ventricular In-flow Tract.
LVOT : Left Ventricular Outflow Tract.
LVP : Lysin-Vasopressin.
LVPSP : Left Ventricular Peak Systolic Pressure.
LVPW : Left Ventricular Posterior Wall.
LVRS : Lung Volume Reduction Surgery.

LVSWI   : Left Ventricular Stroke Work Index.

LW   : Labour Ward.

LZ   : Lower Zone. m **(mm)**   : Muscle(s). (USA).

M   : Male
               Malignant
               Mitosis.

MA   : Marketing Authorization (Application). (USA).
               Maximum Amplitude.
               Mental Age.
               Microalbuminuria.
               Mean Acceleration.

MAA   : Micro-Aggregates of Albumin.

MAbs   : Monoclonal Antibodies. (Ref. IgGI molecules).

MABC   : Motor Assessment Battery for Children.(Ref. motor
               function test in children).

MABP   : Mean Arterial Blood Pressure.

MAC   : Membrane Attack Complex.
               Mid-Arm Circumference.
               Migration Advisory Committee.
               Minimum Alveolar Concentration.
               Monitored Anesthesia Care. (USA).
               Mycobacterium Avium (Complex).

MACE   : Major Adverse Cardiac Event.

MAD   : MaximumAccumulated Dose.
               Mean Absolute Difference.

MADPE   : Median Absolute Performance Error.

MADRS   : Montegomery and Asberg Depression Rating Scale.

MAG   : Malnutrition Advisory Group.
               Myelin-Associated Antibodies.
               Myelin-Associated Glycoprotein

MAG-3   : Mercaptoacetyl Triglycine.

MAGE   : Medical Aid to Galle and Environs. (Ref. Cleft lip/palate
               repair charity).

MAGPI   : Meatal Advancement and Glanduloplasty.

MAHA   : Microangiopathic Haemolytic Anaemia.

MAI	: Mycobacterium Avium-Intracellulare. (Ref. in **HIV** and **AIDS** Patients).
MAIC	: Mycobacterium Avium Intracellulare.
MAIPA	: Monoclonal Antibody Immobilisation of Platelet Antigens.
MAL	: Mid-Axillary Line.
MALT	: Mucosa-Associated Lymphoid Tissue.
MAMC	: Mid-Arm Muscle Circumference.
Mane	: In the Morning.
MANOVA	: Multivariate Analysis of Variance. (Ref. in Statistics).
MAO	: Mono-Amine Oxidase.
MAOIs	: Mono-Amine Oxidase Inhibitors.
MAP	: Mean Airway Pressure.
	Mean Arterial Pressure.
MAPK	: Mitogen-Activated Protein Kinase.
MAPPA	: Multi-Agency Public Protection Arrangements.
MAR	: Missing At Random (Data).
	Mixed Antibody Reaction.
MARS	: Molecular Adsorbents Recirculating System.
MAS	: McCune-Albright Syndrome.
	Meconium Aspiration Syndrome.
	Milk Alkali Syndrome.
MASC	: Medical Academic Science Committee.
MASS	: Multicentre Aneurysm Screening.
MAST	: Medical Anti-Shock Trouser.
	Michigan Alcoholism Screening Test. (USA).
MAT	: Multifocal Atrial Tachycardia.
MAX (max)	: Maximum.
	Maxillar (or Maxillary).
MBC	: Minimal Bacterial Concentration.
MBD	: Metabolic Bone Disease.
MBL	: Mannose-Binding Lectin.
	Menstrual Blood Loss.
MBN	: Multiple Breath Nitrogen (Washout).
MC	: Mast Cells.
	Metacarpal.

	Mesenchymal Chondrosarcoma.
	Monochorionic (Twins).
MCA	: Medicines Control Agency. (Now under **MHRA**).
	Middle Cerebral Artery.
MCAFV	: Middle Cerebral Artery Flow Velocity.
MCCD	: Medical Certificate of Cause of Death.
MCD	: Meningococcal Disease.
	Minimal Change Disease.
MCDK	: Multicystic Dysplastic Kidneys.
MCF	: Maximum Clot Firmness.
MCGN	: Mesangio-Capillary Glomerulonephritis.
MCH	: Mean Cell Haemoglobin.
	Mean Corpuscular Haemoglobin.
MCHC	: Mean Cell Haemoglobin Concentration.
	Mean Corpuscular Haemoglobin Concentration.
MCI	: Mild (or Minimal) Cognitive Impairment.
MCL	: Medial Collateral Ligament.
	Mid-Clavicular Line.
MCLS	: Modified Cormack and Lehane Score (or Grade).
MCN	: Managed Clinical Networks.
	Minimal Change Nephropathy.
	Minocycline.
MCO	: Managed Care Organisation.
MCP	: Metacarpophalangeal.
MCP-1	: Monocyte Chemoattractant Protein 1
MCPJ	: Metacarpal Phalangeal Joint.
MCOs	: Managed Care Organizations. (USA).
MCQ	: Multiple Choice Questions.
MC& S	: Microscopy, Culture and Sensitivity.
MCS	: Multiple Component System.(Ref. version of Haemonetics system).
M-CSF	: Macrophage Colony Stimulating Factor.
MCSS	: Multiple Chemical Sensitivity Syndrome. (Ref. now called Idiopathic Environmental Intolerance Syndrome; **IEIS**).
MCT	: Medium Chain Triglyceride.
MCTD	: Mixed Connective Tissue Disease.
MCU	: Micturating Cysto-urethrography.

MCUG : Micturating Cysto-Urethrogram.
MCV : Mean Cell Volume (or Mean Corpuscular Volume).
MCW : Maternity and Child Welfare.

MD : Malondialdehyde.(Ref. metabolite of free radical-induced Peroxide).
Medical Device.
Medical Doctor. (Doctor of Medicine.)
Mesangial Deposit. (Ref. occurring in Glomerulonephritis).
Microdialysis.
Muscular Dystrophy.
MDA : Malondialdehyde. (Ref. an Assay of free-radicals in Cardiac Disease).
Medical Devices Agency.
Microdialysis Analyser.
MDCT : Multi-Detector Computed Tomography.
MDD : Major Depressive Disorder.
MDDUS : Medical and Dental Defence Union of Scotland.
MDF : Maddery Discriminant Function. (USA).
MDI : Mental Development Index.
Metered-Dose Inhaler.
MDM : Mid-Diastolic Murmur.
MDMA : 3-4-Methylenedioxymethamphetamine. (Ectacy).
MDN : Mean Dilution Number. (Ref. a measurement of ventricular distribution).
MDP : Methylene Diphosphonate. (Ref. in Bone Scanning).
MDPE : Median Prediction Error.
MDR : Multi-Drug Resistant.
MDRD : Modification of Diet in Renal Disease.
MDRTB : Multi-Drug Resistant Tuberculosis. (Ref. Nasocomially-acquired).
MDS : Minimum Data Set.
Myelodysplastic Syndrome.(Ref. a Group of Clonal Haematopoietic Disorders which may progress to Leukaemia).
MDT : Multi-disciplinary Team.
MDTC : Mersey Drug Training and Information Centre. (U.K).

MDTF	: Medium Dose Tissue Factor.
MDU	: Medical Defence Union.
ME	: Myalgic Encephalomyelitis.
MEAMS	: Middlesex Elderly Assessment of Mental State.
MEC	: Median Effective Concentrate.
	Medical Eligibility Criteria.
MECCA	: Medical Errors and Complications.
Med.	: Medicine or Medical.
MED–50	: Median Effective Dose in 50% (of subjects.)
MEE	: Medical Education England.(Ref. oversees medical education and training).
MEF	: Median Edge Frequency.
	Minimal Enteral Feeding.
MEG	: Magnetoencephalogram.
	Magneto-Encephalography.
MELAS	: Mitochondrial Encephalopathy, Lactic Acidosis, Stroke-like episodes Syndrome.
MELD	: Model for End-Stage Liver Disease.
MEN	: Multiple Endocrine Neoplasia..(Ref. Werner`s and Sipple`s syndromes).
MEOS	: Microsomal Ethanol-oxidising System.
MEP	: Motor Evoked Potential.
MEPA	: Managing Emergencies in Paediatric Anaesthesia.
MEPPs	: Miniature End Plate Potentials. (Ref. effects of Neuromuscular blockers).
m**Eq**	: Milli-Equivalent.
MERFF	: Myoclonic Epilepsy with ragged red Fibres (Syndrome.): (Ref. Myoclonic Epilepsy with cerebral ataxia, dementia, deafness, and optical atrophy).
MESA	: Microsurgical Sperm Aspiration.
MET	: Medical Emergency Team. (Ref. for identification of high risk patients).
	Meta-analysis.
met**Hb**	: Met-Haemoglobin.
MetS	: Metabolic Syndrome.(Ref. combination of; cardiovascular disease, Insulin Resistance; Glucose intolerance and increased Free Fatty Acids).

METS	: Metabolic Equivalents.
MEWS	: Modified Early Warning Score.(Ref. Paediatric early warning aggregate Score).
MF	: Multifactorial.
	Mycosis Fungoides.
MFDS	: Maxillofacial and Dental Surgery.
MFE	: Medicine for the Elderly.
MFET	: Medical Fair and Ethical Trade.
MFH	: Malignant Fibro-Histiocytoma.
MFI	: Mean Fluorescence Intensity.
MFPR	: Multi-Foetal Pregnancy Reduction.
MFS	: Marfan Syndrome.
MFV	: Mean Flow Velocity.
mg	: Milligrams.
Mg++	: Magnesium.
MG	: Myasthenia Gravis.
M3G	: Morphine-3-Glucuronide.
M6G	: Morphine-6-Gluculonide.
MGMT	: O-Methylguanine Methyltransferase (Ref. **DNA**).
MGN	: Membranous Glomerulonephritis.
MGPS	: Multi-Item Gamma Poisson Shrinker. (USA).
MGUS	: Monoclonal Gammaopathy of Undetermined Significance.
MH	: Malignant Hyperpyrexia (or Hyperthermia).
MHA	: Mental Health Act.
MHAC	: Mental Health Act Commission.
MHC	: Major Histocompatibility Complex (Deficiency).
MHE	: Malignant Hyperpyrexia Equivalent.
MHI	: Manual Hyper-inflation.
MHMDS	: Mental Health Minimum Dataset.
MHN	: Malignant Hyperpyrexia Normal.
MHNM	: Malignant Hyperpyrexia Normal Muscle.
MHO	: Medical Health Officer.
MHOA	: Mental Health in Old Age.
MHOS	: Mental Health Outreach Service.

MHRA	: Medicines and Healthcare Products Regulatory Agency (or Authority).
MHRT	: Mental Health Review Tribunal.
MHS	: Malignant Hyperpyrexia Susceptible.
MHSM	: Malignant Hyperpyrexia Susceptible Muscle.
MHSW	: Management of Health and Safety at Work.
MHU	: Mental Health Unit.
MI	: Mental Illness.
	Mentally Impaired.
	Mitral Incompetence (or Insufficiency).
	Myocardial Infarct (or Infarction).
	Myocardial Ischaemia.
MIB	: Metaiodobenzylguanidine.
MIBG	: Meta-Iodo-benzylguanidine (Imaging).
MIC	: Minimum Inhibitory Concentration. (Ref. antibiotic concentration to inhibit microbio-growth).
MI & D	: Mentally Ill and Dangerous.
MIF	: Melanocyte-Inhibiting.
	Migration-Inhibitor Factor.
MIGET	: Multiple Inert Gas Elimination Technique.
MILS	: Manual In-line Stabilisation. (Ref. in cervical spine injuries management).
MIMS	: Monthly Index of Medical Specialities.
Min (min)	: Minute/s.
Min-Cex	: Mini-Clinical Evaluation Exercise.
MIP	: Maximum Inspiratory Pressure.
	Maximum Intensity Projection. (Ref. **CT** imaging).
MIRACLE	**:** Multicentre Insync Randomised Clinical Evaluation.
MIS	: Minimum Invasive Surgery.
	Mullerian-Inhibiting Substance.
Misc.	: Miscarriage.
MIST	: Mechanism, Injury, Signs and Symptoms, and Treatment.
MIT	: Medial Infraclavicular Technique.(Ref. Brachial Plexus Block Technique).
Mj	: Megajoules.

mL (ml)	: Millilitre.
MLAC	: Minimum Local Anaesthetic (Analgesic) Concentration.
MLAEP	: Mid-Latency Auditory-Evoked Potential.
MLB	: Microlaryngoscopy and Bronchoscopy.
MLCF	: Medical Leadership Competency Framework.
MLD	: Metachromatic Leucodystrophy.
MLF	: Medial Longitudinal Fasciculus.
MLP	: Multi-layer Perception.
MLR	: Medical Loss Ratio.(Percentage of Total Cost to Total Revenue). (USA).
	Middle Latency Response.
mm.	: Millimetre/s
MM	: Malignant Melanoma.
	Multiple Myloma.
M&M	: Morbidity and Mortality.
MMA	: Maxillo-Mandibular Advancement.
	Methylmalonic Acid.
	Middle Meatal Antrostomy.
MMC	: Migrating Motility Complex.
	Modernising Medical Careers.
MMCPT	: Modernising Medical Careers Programme Team.
MMD	: Mass Median Diameter. (Ref. particle size in Anaesthetic circuit Filters).
MMF	: Mycophenolate Mofetil.
MMG	: Mechanomyography.(Ref a test for post-operative recuralisation; **PORC**).
mmH2O	: Millimetres of Water.
mmHq	: Millimetres of Mercury.
mmols	: Millimoles.
MMM	: Mitozantrone, Methotraxate, Mitomycin C.
MMPs	: Matrix Metallo-Proteinases.(Ref. extracellular endopeptides in Homeostasis).
MMPA	: Maxillary Mandibular Planes Angle.
MMR	: Mass Miniature Radiography.
	Measles, Mumps and Rubella (vaccine).
	Mismatch Genetic Repair.
MMRV	: Measles; mumps; Rubella Vaccine.
MMSE	: Mini-Mental State Examination (Score).

MMT	: Machine Market Test.
	Mixed Mullerian Tumour.
MMV	: Medicines for Malaria Venture.
Mn	: Manganese.
MN	: Membranous Nephropathy.
MND	: Motor Neurone Disease.
MNOE	: Malignant Necrotising Otitis Externa.
MO	: Medical Officer.
Mo	: Molybdenum.
MoAbs	: Monoclonal Antibodies.
MOAS	: Modified Overt Aggression Scale.
MODS	: Multi-Organ Dysfunction Syndrome.
MODY	: Maturity-Onset Diabetes of the Young.
MOEH	: Medical Officer for Environmental Health.
MOF	: Multi-Organ Failure.
MOFIT	: Multiple Out Fracture of the Inferior Turbinate.
MOH	: Medication Overuse Headache.(Ref.Headache due to overuse of analgesics).
	Medical Officer of Health.
Mol	: Mole.
MOM (MoM)	: Milk of Magnesia.
	Multiples of the Median.
MONA	: Morphine, Oxygen, Nitroglycerine, Aspirin.
MONICA	: Monitoring Trends and determinants in Cardiovascular Disease.
MOP	: Medical Out-Patient.
	Mew-Opioid Protein(Receptor). (Ref.analgesic and respiratory depression).
MOR	: Mew-Opioid Receptor.
MORE	: Multiple Outcomes of Raloxifene Evaluation.
mOsmol	: Milliosmols.
MOST	: Multi-Centre Osteoarthritis Study.
MPA	: Management Professional Activity.
	Medroxyprogesterone Acetate.
	Microscopic Polyangitis.

MPAA   : Male Pattern Androgenic Alopecia.
MPAP   : Mean Pulmonary Arterial Pressure.
MPD   : Maximum Permissible Dose.
                 Multiple Personality Disorder.
                 Myeloproliferative Disease.
                 Myofacial Pain Dysfunction.
MPET   : Multi-Professional Education and Training.
MPGN   : Membrano-Prolifirative Glomerulonephritis.
MPH   : Massive Pulmonary Haemorrhage.
MPHR   : Maximum Predicted Heart Rate.
MPI   : Master Patient Index.
                 Myocardial Perfusion Imaging.
MPIG   : Minimum Practice Income Guarantee.
MPLT   : Modified Pressure Leak Test.
MPM   : Mortality Probability Model.
MPN   : Microscopic Polyangiitis Nodosa.
MPOs   : Myleoperoxidases.(Ref. cytoplasmic enzymes used in
                 ANA testing).
MPPS   : Medicare Prospective Payment System. (USA).
MPQ   : McGill Pain Questionnaire.
MPS   : Macular Photocoagulation Study.
                 Medical Protection Society.
                 Mucopolysaccharidosis.
MPTP   : Methyl-Phenyl-Tetrahydro-Pyridine.
MPU   : Medical Practitioners Union.
MPV   : Mean Platelet Volume.

MR(m/r)   : Modified Release.
MR   : Magnetic Resonance.
                 Manual Removal.
                 Mental Retardation.
                 Mitral Regurgitation (or Insufficiency).
MRA   : Magnetic Resonance Angiography.
MRC   : Magnetic Resonance Cholangiography.
                 Medical Research Council.
MRCNS   : Multiple-Resistant Coagulase-Negative Staphylococcus.
MRCOG   : Member of the Royal College of Obstetrics and
                 Gynaecology.

MRCP	: Magnetic Resonance Cholangio-Pancreatography.
	Member of the Royal College of Physicians.
MRCPsych.	: Member of the Royal College of Psychiatrists.
MRCPCH	: Member of the Royal College of Paediatrics and Child Health.
MRCS	: Member of the Royal College of Surgeons.
MRD	: Minimal Residual Disease.
MRI	: Magnetic Resonance Imaging.
MRKH	: Mayer-Rokitansky Kuster Houser (Syndrome).
MRM	: Modified Radical Mastoidectomy.
mRNA	: Messenger Ribonucleic Acid.
MRND	: Modified Radical Neck Dissection
MRP	: Mandibular Reconstruction Plate.
	Mutual Recognition Procedure. (USA).
MRS	: Magnetic Resonance Spectroscopy.
MRSA	: Methicillin-Resistant Staphylococcus aureus.
MRSS	: Morningside Rehabilitation Status Scale.
MRU	: Mass Radiography Unit.
MS	: Maternal Serum.
	Morphine Sulphate.
	Multiple Scelerosis.
	Mitral Stenosis.
	Musculoskeletal.
MSA	: Multisystem Atrophy.
MSAF	: Meconium-Stained Amniotic Fluid.
MSAFP (MS-AFP)	: Maternal Serum-Alpha-Foetoprotein Test.
MSc	: Master of Science.
MSC	: Medical Schools Council.
	Medical Students Committee.
	Musculoskeletal Conditions.
MSD	: Mark Sharp and Dhome.
MSDS	: Material Safety Data Sheets. (USA).
MSE	: Mental State Examination.
MSF	: Medicius Sans Frontieres.
	Multisource Feedback.
MSG	: Management Steering Group.
	Monosodium Glutamate.

MSH	: Melanocyte-Stimulating Hormone.
MSK	: Medullary Sponge Kidney.
MSL	: Meconium Stained Liquor.
	Medical Science Liaison (Function). (USA).
	Multiple Symmetric Lipomatosis.
MSLT	: Multiple Sleep Latency Test.
MSM	: Men(who have) Sex with Men.
	Monosodium Urate Monohydrate.
MSN	: Medial Septal Nucleus. (Ref. a cerebral structure).
MSNA	: Muscular Sympathetic Nerve Activity.
MSbP	: Manchausen Syndrome by Proxy.
MSS	: Montegomery Schizophrenia Scale.
MSSA	: Meticillin Susceptible Staphylococcus aureus.
MST	: Morphine Sulphate (Slow Release).
	Multisystem Therapy.
MSU	: Mid Stream Specimen of Urine.
MSUD	: Maple Syrup Urine Disease.
MSW	: Medical Social Worker.
MT	: Manual Techniques.
	Metatarsal.
	Midwifery Teacher.
MTA (MeTA)	: Medicines Transparency Alliance. (Ref. International Organisation dealing with **WHO** and World Bank on Drugs quality; availability; affordability; for the poor populations of the World).
MTA	: Mineral Trioxide (Aggregate).
MTAS	: Medical Training and Application Service.
MTC	: Medullary Thyroid Carcinoma.
MTCD	: Mixed Connective Tissue Disease.
MTCT	: Mother to Child Transmission.
MTD	: Midwife Teachers` Diploma.
	Multidisciplinary Team.
MTFC	: Multi-dimensional Intervention Foster Care.
mth/s	: Month/s.
MTHFR	: Methyltetrahydrofolate Reductase.
MTP	: Massive (Blood) Transfusion Protocol.
MTPJ	: Metartasal Phalangeal Joint.

MTT	: Mean Transit Time.
MTX	: Methotrexate.
MUA	: Manipulation Under Anaesthesia.
MUAC	: Mid Upper Arm Circumference.
MUD	: Matched Unrelated Donor (Transplant).
MUFA	: Mono Unsaturated Fatty Acids.
MUPs	: Motor Unit Potentials.
MUS	: Medically Unexplained Symptoms.
MUST	: Malnutrition Universal Screening Tool.
MUSTIC	: Multisite Pacing in Intraventricular Conduction Delay.
MV	: Mechanical Ventilation.
	Minimum Ventilation.
	Minute Volume. (see under **MVol.**).
	Mitral Valve.
MVol	: Minute Volume. (Ref. during Ventilation).
MVA	: Mannual Vacuum Aspiration.
	Mitral Valve Area.
MVP	: Mitral Valve Prolapse.
MVR	: Mitral Valve Replacement.
MVT	: Monomorphic Ventricular Tachycardia.
MWM	: Mobilisation with Movement.
MWO	: Mental Welfare Officer.
M-XR	: Mass X-ray.
MZ	: Middle Zone.
	Monozygous or Monozygotic (Twins).
N (nl)	: Normal.
	Number of Sample size.
N₂	: Nitrogen.
Na+	: Sodium.
NA	: Narcotics Anonymous.
	Negative Affectivity.
	Noradrenaline.

Not Applicable.

Nurse Anaesthetist.

Nursing Auxillary.

NAATs (NATs): Nucleic Acid Amplification Tests.

NABQI   : N-Acetyl-benzoquinoneimine.

NAC   : N-acetyl cystine. (Ref. in Acute Renal Failure).

National Asthma Campaign.

NACC   : National Association for Colitis and Crohn's Disease.

NACL (NaCl) : Sodium Chloride.

NACNE   : National Advisory Committee on Nutrition Education.

NACS   : Neurologic and Adaptive Capacity.(Ref. measurement of Neonatal status at birth).

NAD   : Nicotinamide Adenine Dinucleotide.

No Abnormality Detected (or Nothing abnormal detected).

No Apparent Disease.

NADP   : Nicotinamide Adenine Phosphate.

NADR   : National **AIDS** Development Research.

NAFLD   : Non-Alcoholic Fatty Liver Disease.

NAI   : Non-Accidental Injury.

NAIT   : Neonatal Alloimmune Thrombocytopenia.

NAMCW   : National Association for Maternal and Child Welfare.

NAME(S)   : Nevi, Atrial myxoma, Myxoid neurofibromas, Ephelides(frekles) Syndrome.

NAMH   : National Association for Mental Health.

NANB   : Non-A, Non-B (Hepatitis C).

NANC   : Non-Adrenergic, Non-Cholinergic Nerves.

NAO   : National Audit Office.

NaOH   : Sodium Hydroxide.

NAP   : Neutrophil Alkaline Phosphatase.

NAPPG   : National Association for Patient Participation Groups.

NAPNA   : N-Nitro-arginine P-Nitro-anilide. (Ref. a non-specific inhibitor of Nitric Oxide synthatases.)

NAPQI   : N-Acetyl-P-benzoquinoneimine.

NARES   : Non-Allergic Rhinitis with Eosinophilia.

NARI   : Noradrenaline Re-uptake Inhibitor.

NAS   : No Added Salt.

NASBA   : Nucleic Acid Sequence-based Amplification.

NASC	: National Anaesthesia Society`s Committee.
NASCET	: North American Symptomatic Carotid Endarterectomy Trial.
NASGPs	: National Association of Sessional General Practitioners.
NASH	: Non-Alcoholic Steatohepatitis.
NaSSA	: Noradrenaline and Specific Serotonin Antagonist.
NATN	: National Association of Theatre Nurses.
NatPaCT	: National Primary and Care Trust (Development Programme).
N & V	: Nausea and Vomiting.
NAWCH	: National Association for the Welfare of Children in Hospital.
NBA	: National Blood Authority.
NBAP	: National Booked Admissions Programme.
NBI	: National Beds Enquiry.
	No Bone Injury.
NBM	: Nil by Mouth.
	Nucleus Basalis of Meynert. (Ref. a Brain structure).
NBT	: Nitroblue Tetrazolium Reduction Test.
NBTV	: Non-Bacterial Thrombotic Vegetation.
NC	: Nasal Catheter.
	Nuclear Cardiology.
NCA	: Nurse Controlled Analgesia.
	National Clinical Audit.
NCAA	: National Clinical Assessment Authority.
NCAAG	: National Clinical Audit Advisory Group.
NCAS	: National Clinical Assessment Service.
NCASP	: National Clinical Audit Support Programme.
NCCC	: Northern Centre for Cancer Care.
NCCU	: Neuro-Critical Care Unit.
NCCMERP	: National Co-ordinating Council for Medication Error Reporting and Prevention.
NCD	: Nutrition-related Chronic Disease.
NCDs	: Non-Communicable Diseases.
NCE	: National Confidential Enquiry.

NCEPOD : National Confidential Enquiry into Patient Outcome and Death.

NCG : National Commissioning Group.

NCGC : National Clinical Guideline Centre.

NCGC-AC : National Clinical Guideline Centre-Acute and Chronic Conditions.

NCHS : National Centre for Health Statistics.

NCHSPCS : National Council for Hospice and Specialist Palliative Care Services.

NCL : No Cautionary Labels.

NCMRR : National Centre for Medical Rehabilitation Research.

NCPC : National Council for Palliative Care.

NCPP : Nasal Continuous Positive Pressure.

NCR : National Care Record.

NCRN : National Cancer Research Network.

NCS : National Care Services.
Nerve Conduction Studies.

NCSC : National Care Standards Commission.

NCSE : Non-Convulsive Status Epilepticus.

NCSP : National Clamydia Screening Programme.

NCT : National Childbirth Trust.

NCVs : Nerve Conduction Velocities.

NCVM : Non-Compaction of the Ventricular Myocardium.

NCX : Electrogenic Sodium /Calcium exchanger.(Ref. calcium myocardial pathway).

ND : Normal Delivery.
Not Diagnosed.
Not Done.
Notifiable Disease.

NDA : National Diebetes Audit.
National Institute on Drug Abuse.
New Drug Application. (USA).

NDN(C) : National District Nurse Certificate.

NDNS : National Diet and Nutrition Survey.

NDTMS : National Drugs Treatment Monitoring System.

NE : Norepinephrine.

	Not Enlarged.
NEAT	: Non-Exercise Activity Thermogenesis.
NEB (Neb)	: Nebulised/Nebuliser.
NEC	: Necrotising Entero-Colitis (or Enterococci).
NECN	: North of England Cancer Network.
NED	: Neuro-Evoked Depth.
NEJM	: New England Journal of Medicine.
NeLH	: National Electronic Library for Health.
NEMO	: Nano-based Capsule Endoscopy.(Ref. molecular imaging and Optical biopsy).
NeP	: Neuropathic Pain.
NEP	: Nucleotide Excision Pathway.
NES	: **NHS** Education (for Scotland).
NET-EN	: Norethisterone Oenanthate.
NETs	: Neuro-Endocrine Tumours.
NEURO	: Neurology.
Neut.	: Neutrophilis.
NEXUS	: National Emergency X-Radiography Utilisation Study.
NF	: Neurofibromatosis.
	Necrotising Faciatis.
NFA	: Near Fatal Asthma (Attack).
	No Further Action.
NFCIs	: Non-Freezing Cold Injuries.
NFP	: Natural Family Planning.
	Net Filtration Pressure.
NFR	: Not for Resuscitation.
	Nurses for Reform.
NFS	: National Food Survey.
NFSC	: Number of Fluctuations per Second.(Ref. parameter of skin conductance).
NFT	: Nuchal Fold Translucency.
NFV	: No Further Visit.
ng	: Nanogram.
NG	: Nasogastric.
	Neoplastic Growth.
	New Growth.
NGASR	: Nurses Global Assessment of Suicide Risk.

NGF	: Nerve Growth Factor.
nGMS	: New General Medical Services (Contract).
NGO	: Non-Government Agency.
NGRS	: Numbered Graphic Rating Scale. (Ref. in Statistics and Validation).
NGT	: Nasogastric Tube.
NGU	: Non-Gonococcal Urethritis.

NH₃	: Ammonia.
NHANES	: National Health and Nutrition Examination Survey.
NHB	: Non-Heart Beating (Organ.)
NHBD	: Non-Heart Beating Donation.
NHBOD	: Non-Heart Beating Organ Donor.
NHC	: National Hospice Council.
NHI	: National Health Insurance.
NHL	: Non-Hodgkin Lymphoma.
NHMRC	: National Health and Medical Research Council.
NHP	: Nottingham Health Profile.
NHS	: National Health Service.
NHSC	: National Health Service Confederation.
NHSCRD	: National Health Service Centre for Reviews and Dissemination.
NHSE	: National Health Service Employee. National Health Service Executive.
NHSI	: National Health Service Institute (for Innovation and Improvement).
NHSIA	: National Health Service Information Authority.
NHSL	: National Health Service Logistics.
NHSLA	: National Health Service Litigation Authority.
NHS-LIFT	: National Health Service Local Improvement Finance Trust.
NHS-QIS	: National Health Service Quality Improvement (for Scotland).
NHSRF	: National Health Service Retirement Fellowship.
NHST	: National Health Service Trust.

Ni	: Nickel.
NIAA	: National Institute of Academic Anaesthesia.

NIACE	: National Institute of Adult Continuing Education.
NIAID	: National Institute of Allergy and Infectious Diseases.
NIBP	: Non-Invasive Blood Pressure.
NICE	: National Institute for Health and Clinical Excellence (or National Institute for Clinical Excellency).
NICEIP	: National Institute for Health and Clinical Excellence International Procedures (Programme).
NICO	: Neuralgia-Inducing Cavitational Osteonecrosis.
NICU	: Neonatal Intensive Care Unit. Neuro-Intensive Care Unit.
NIDDM	: Non-Insulin Dependent Diabetes Mellitus.
NIDMD	: Northern Ireland Drug Misuse Database.
NIH	: National Institute of Health.
NIHL	: Noise-Induced Hearing Loss.
NIHR	: National Institute for Health Research.
NIHRTC	: National Institute for Health Research`s Trainees Co-ordinating Centre.
NIL	: Not in Labour.
NIMHE	: National Institute for Mental Health in England.
NINB	: Northern Irish National Board for Nursing.
NINDS	: National Institute of Neurological Disorders and Stroke.
NIOSH	: National Institute of Occupational Safety and Health. (Ref. in the **USA**).
NIPPV	: Nasal Intermittent Positive Pressure Ventilation Non-Invasive Positive Pressure Ventilation.
NIPS	: Neonatal Infant Pain Scale.
NIRS	: Near-Infrared Spectroscopy.
NISS	: New Injury Severity Score.
NIV	: Non-Invasive Ventilation.
NJ	: Nasojejunal (Feeding Tube.)
NK	: Natural Killer. (Ref. in altered immune reaction). Not Known.
NKCC	: Natural Killer Cell Cytotoxicity.
NKF	: National Kidney Foundation.
NKH	: Non-Ketotic Hyperosmolar (states).

NLD	: Necrobiosis Lipoidica Diabeticorum.
NLIAH	: National Leadership and Innovation Agency for Healthcare (in Wales).
NLP	: Neuro Linguistic Programming.(Ref. in Negative Emotional Partners).
NLR	: Negative Likelihood Ratio.
NLS	: Neonatal Life Support.
NLST	: National Lung Screening Trial.

NM	: Neuro-muscular.
NMC	: Nursing and Midwifery Council.
NMDA	: N-Methyl-D-Aspartate(blocker).(Ref. receptor-mediated hyperexcitability).
NMDP	: National Marrow Donor Program. (USA).
NMJ	: Neuro-Muscular Junction.
NMN	: N-methylnicotinamide.
NMR	: Nuclear Magnetic Resonance (Imaging).
NMRS	: Nuclear Magnetic Resonance Spectroscopy.
NMS	: Neuroleptic Malignant Syndrome. (Ref. related to Bradykinesia). New Mobility Score.
NMT	: Neuro-Muscular Transmission.

NND	: Neonatal Death.
NNF	: Number Needed to Follow.
NNH	: Number Needed to Harm. (Ref. in Adverse outcomes of Treatment).
NNRTI	: Non-Nucleotide Reverse Transcriptase Inhibitor.
NNT	: Number Needed to Treat.
NNTI	: Non-nucleotide Reverse Transcriptase Inhibitor.
NNU	: Neonatal Unit.

NO	: Nitric Oxide.
N2O	: Nitrous Oxide.
NOAD	: National Obstetric Anaesthesia Database.
NOAH	: Neoadjuvent Herceptin (Study).
NOC	: Nitric Oxide Releasing Compound.

Nocte	: At night.
NOF	: Neck of Femur.
NOFTT	: Non-Organic Failure to Thrive.
NO-MI	: None-O-wave Myocardial Infarct.
NONMEN	: Non-linear Mixed Effects Modelling.
NOP	: Nociceptin (Receptor.)
NOS	: National Osteoporosis Society.
	Nitric Oxide Synthase (or Synthatase).
	Not Otherwise Specified.
NOSIE	: Nurses Observation Scale for In-Person Evaluation.
NOTB	: National Ophthalmic Treatment Board.
NP	: Nasophalangeal.
	Nurse Practitioner.
NPA	: Nasopharyngeal Aspirate.
NPC	: Nasopharyngeal Carcinoma.
	National Prescribing Centre.
nPCR	: Normalised Protein Catabolic Rate.
NPD	: Narcissitic Personality Disorder.
NPEF	: Nurse Prescribers Extended Formulary.
NPEN	: Non-Protein Energy : Nitrogen (Ratio).
NPf IT	: National Programme for Information Technology (in the **NHS**).
NPF	: Nurse Prescribers Formulary.
NPH	: Normal Pressure Hydrocephalus.
NPHS	: National Public Health Service (of Wales).
NPIS	: National Poisons Information Service.
NPMS	: National Psychiatric Morbidity Study.
NPO	: Nihil per os (Ref. Latin for; Nil by mouth).
NPRI	: National Panel for Research Integrity. (USA).
NPS	: Nasal Pharyngeal Stenosis.
	Nottingham Physiology Simulator.
NPSA	: National Patient Safety Agency.
NPT	: Near Patient Testing. (Ref. with regard to **INR** monitoring in homes).
	Nocturnal Penile Tumescence.
NPV	: Negative Pressure Ventilation.

NP-Y : Neuro-Peptide Y.(Ref. in control of
Gonadotrophin-releasing Hormone).

NQMI(nQMI) : Non-Q wave Myocardial Infarction.

NR : Normal Range.
NRAC : (National Health Service Scotland) Resource Allocation
Committee.
NRAG : National Radiotherapy Advisory Group.
NRAS : National Rheumatoid Arthritis Society.
NRBC : Nucleated Red Blood Cells.
NREM : Non-Rapid Eye Movement (sleep).
NRL : Natural Rubber Latex.
NRLS : National Reporting and Learning Services.
NROGPT : National Recruitment Office for General Practice
Training.
NRPB : National Radiological Protection Board.
NRS : Numerical Rating Scale.
NRT : Nicotine Replacement Therapy.
NRTI : Non-nucleoside Reverse Transcriptase Inhibitor.

NS : Nephrotic Syndrome.
Nervous System.
Neurosarcoidosis.
Normal Saline (i.e 0.9% Sodium Chloride).
Not Significant.
NSAIDs : Non-Steroidal Anti-Inflammatory Drugs.
NSCLC : Non-Squamous Cell Lung Cancer.
NSCR : National Summary Care Record.
NSD : Neuro-Sensory Deficit.
NSE : Neonatal Sepsis Evaluation.
Neuron-Specific Enolyse.(Ref. adverse neurological
outcomes following Thoraco-Abdominal Aortic
Aneurysm surgery).
Sodium-Calcium Exchanger.
NSEP : Needle-Syringe-Exchange Programme.
NSF : National Service Framework.
NSHAP : National Social life, Health and Aging Project.

NSHN	: National Self-Harm Network.
NSM	: Nerve-Sheath Myxoma.
NSP	: Non-Starch Polysaccharides.
NSR	: No Sign of Recurrence.
NST	: Non-Shivering Thermogenesis.
	Non-Stress Test.
NSTEACS	: Non-ST segment Elevation Acute Coronary Syndromes.
NSTEMI	: Non-ST Elevated Myocardial Infarction.
NSU	: Non-Specific Urethritis.
NT	: Nuchal Translucency.
	Nurse Teacher.
N&T	: Nose and Throat.
NTA	: National Treatment Agency (for Substance Misuse).
NTB	: Necrotising Tracheobronchitis.
NTCC	: New Technology in Cervical Cancer (Study).
NTDs	: Neural Tube Defects.
NTDS	: North Thames Dialysis Study.
NTI	: Naso-Tracheal Intubation. (Ref. in Anaesthesia).
	Nucleotide reverse-Transcriptase Inhibitor.
NTN	: National Training Number.
NTORS	: National Treatment Outcome Research Study.
NTS	: Nucleus Tractus Solitarius.
NTX	: N-Telopeptides of Type 1 Collagen.
NUMINE	: Network of Users of Microcomputers in Nurse Education.
N&V	: Nausea and Vomiting.
NVD	: Normal Vaginal Delivery.
NVQ	: National Vocational Qualification.
NWBPOP	: Non-weight-bearing Plaster of Paris.
NWMA	: New Wall Motion Abnormalities. (Ref. in Echocardiography).
	New Ways of Working in Anaesthesia.
NXG	: Necrobiosis Xanthogranuloma.

NYD	: Not Yet Diagnosed.
NYHA	: New York Heart Association. (USA).
NYK	: Not Yet Known.

O	: Ovary.
O₂	: Oxygen.
OA	: Occipito-Anterior.
	Oesophageal Atrasia.
	Osteoarthritis.
OAA	: Obstetric Anaesthetists Association.
OAAS	: Observers Assessment of Alertness/Sedation. (USA).
OAB	: Over-Active Bladder.
OAI	: Oleic Acid (Lung) Injury.
OARSI	: Osteoarthritis Research Society.
OAS	: Oral Allergy Syndrome.
	Orbital Apex Syndrome.
OAT	: Occluded Artery Trial.
	Out-of-area Treatment.

OBD	: Organic Brain Disorder.
Obs.	: Observations.
OBS	: Obstetrics.
	Organic Brain Syndrome.
	Output Based Specification.
OBS & GYNAE	: Obstetrics and Gynaecology.

OC	: On-Call.
	Open Cholecystectomy.
OCBs	: Oligoclonal Bands.
OCC	: Oral Cavity Cancer.
OCD	: Obsessive Compulsive Disorder.
	Osteochondritis Dissicans.
OCMO	: Office of the Chief Medical Officer (of Wales).
OCPs	: Oral Contraceptive Pills.
OCP	: Oral Contraceptive Pill.
OCT	: Ornithine Carbamoyltransferase. (Ref. a Urea cycle Disorder).

	Optical Coherence Tomography.
	Oxytocin Challenge Test.
OCTR	: Open Carpal Tunnel Release.
od	: Omni die. (Ref. Latin for; once a day or "every day").
OD	: Observed Difference.
	Oculus dexter (Right Eye).
	Oesophageal Doppler.
	Once Daily.
	Optical Density.
	Overdose.
OD 450	: Optical Density at 450 nm.
ODAs	: Operating Department Assistants.
ODC	: Oxygen Dissociation Curve.
ODD	: Oppositional Defiant Disorder.
ODNs	: Oligodeoxynucleotides. (Ref. used in pain treatment for Allodynia).
ODP	: Operating Department Practitioner..
OE	: Otitis Externa.
O/E (OE)	: On Examination.
OECD	: Organisation for Economic Cooperation and Development.
OEF	: Oxygen Extraction Fraction.
OER	: Oxygen Extraction Ratio.
OFC	: Orbital Frontal Cortex.
	Occipital-Frontal Circumference.
OFCD	: Oculofacial Cardiodental (Syndrome).
OFM	: Oxygen-Flow Modulator.
OFQUAL	: Office of the Qualifications and Examinations Regulator.
OGD	: Oesophago-Gastro-Duodenoscopy.
	Oxygen-Glucose Deprivation.
OGS	: Oxogenic Steroids.
OGTT	: Oral Glucose Tolerance Test.
OH	: Obstetric History.
	Occupational Health.
	Oral Hygiene.

	Orthostatic Hypotension.
OHA	: Oral Hypoglycaemic Agent.
	Oxford Handbook of Anaesthesia.
OHAM	: Oxford Handbook of Acute Medicine.
OHCA	: Out of Hospital Cardiac Arrest.
OHCC	: Oxford Handbook of Critical Care.
OHCLI	: Oxford Handbook of Clinical and Laboratory Investigation
OHCM	: Oxford Handbook of Clinical Medicine.
OHCS	: Oxford Handbook of Clinical Specialities.
OHE	: Office of Health Economics.
OHEM	: Oxford Handbook of Emergency Medicine.
OHGP	: Oxford Handbook of General Practice.
OHI	: Oral Hygiene Instructions.
OHN	: Occupational Health Nursing.
OHNC	: Occupational Health Nursing Certificate.
OHOG	: Oxford Handbook of Obstetrics and Gynaecology.
OHPA	: Office of the Health Professions Adjudicator.
OHS	: Obesity-Hyperventilation Syndrome.
OHSC	: Occupational Health Smart Card.
OHSS	: Ovarian Hyperstimulation Syndrome.
OHTP	: Out of Hospital Transfusion Program. (USA).
OI	: Osteogenesis Imperfecta.
OIs	: Opportunistic Infections.
OLT	: Orthotopic Liver Transplantation.
OLV	: One Lung Ventilation.
OM (o.m)	: Omni mane. (Ref. Latin for; "every morning").
OM	: Osteomyelitis
	Otitis Media.
OMC	: Osteomeatal Complex.
OME	: Otitis Media with Effusion.
OMERACT	: Outcome Measures in Rheumatology Clinical Trials.
OMIM	: Online Mendelian Inheritance in Man (Database).
OMIT	: Ocular Microtremor. (Ref. physiological eye tremor depressed by Propofol Aneasthesia).

OMP	: Oral Medicine and Pathology.
OMS	: Oral and Maxillofacial Surgeons.
OMV	: Oxford Miniature Veporiser.
ON (o.n)	: Omni nocte. (Ref. Latin for; "every night").
ONC	: Orthopaedic Nurses` Certificate.
OND	: Ophthalmic Nursing Diploma.
ONDCP	: Office of Narcotic Drug Control Policy.
ONJ	: Osteo-Necrosis of the Jaw.
ONS	: Office of National Statistics.
OOB	: Out of Bed.
OOH	: Out-of-Hours.
OOPE	: Out of Programme Experience.(Ref. experienced applicants for training).
OORR	: On-line Orders and Results Reporting.
OP	: Occipito-Posterior.
	Operation.
	Oropharyngeal
	Out-Patients.
O & P	: Ova and Parasites.
OPA	: Out-Patient Appointment.
OPCAB	: Off-Pump Coronary Artery Grafting (or Bypass).
OPD	: Out-Patients Department.
OPG	: Orthopantomogram.
	Osteoprotegerin.(Ref. **RANK receptor** activation remodelling in Bone).
OPLL	: Ossification of the Posterior Longitudinal Ligament.
OPS	: Objective Pain Scale.
	Orthogonal Polarisation Spectral. (Ref. an Imaging technique).
OPSI	: Overwhelming Post-Splenectomy Infection.
OPT	: Orthopantomogram.
OPTIMAL	: Outpatient Physical Therapy Improvement in Movement Assessment.
OPV	: Oral Polio Vaccine.

OR : Odds Ratio.
Operating Room.
ORBIT : Outcome Reporting Bias in Trials.
ORCON : Operational Resaerch Consultants.
ORI : Office of Research Integrity. (USA).
ORIF : Open Reduction and Internal Fixation.
ORh-ve : Blood Group O, Rhesus Negative.
ORS : Oral Rehydration Solutions.
ORT : Oral Re-hydration Therapy.
ORTHO : Orthopaedics.

OS : Oculus sinister (Left Eye).
OSA : Obstructive Sleep Apnoea.
OSAS : Obstructive Sleep Apnoea Syndrome.
OSCAR : Organisation for Sickle Cell Anaemia Research.
Optimising Surgical Care and Assessment.
OSCE : Objective Structured Clinical Examination.
OSI : Open System Interconnection.
Osmol : Osmoles.
OSP : Oncocytic Schneiderian Papilloma.

OT : Occupational Therapy (or Occupational Therapist).
Occipito-Transverse.
Old Tuberculin.
OTC : Over-the-Counter.
Ornithine Transcarbarmylase (Enzyme).
OTFC : Oral Transmucosal Fentanyl Citrate.

OU : Oculi unitas (Both Eyes).

OVD : Occlusion Vertical Dimension.

OXVASC : Oxford Vascular Study.(Ref. Study in acute vascular events or **TIAs**).

P : Pharmacy (only medicine). (USA).
Phosphorus.
Pubic.

	Pulse.
P₂	: Pulmonary second Heart Sound.
PA	: Patients Association.
	Pernicious Anaemia.
	Postero-Anterior.
	Pressure Area.
	Professional Activity.
	Pulmonary Angiogram.
	Pulmonary Artery.
	Physical Activity.
P/A	: Per Abdomen.
PA(rt-PA)	:(recombinant tissue) Plasminogen Activator.(Ref. in acute ischaemic stroke)
PABA	: Para-Aminobenzoic Acid.
PABD	: Preoperative Autologous Blood Donation.
PAC	: Pulmonary Artery Catheter.
	Premature Atrial Contraction.
PACA	: Professionals Against Child Abuse.
PACES	**:** Practical Assessment and Clinical Examinations.(Ref. e.g **MRCP** Examination)
PACI	: Partial Anterior Circulation Infarct.
PaCO₂	: Partial pressure of Carbon Dioxide (in arterial blood).
PACS	: Partial Anterior Circulation Stroke.
	Picture Archiving and Communications Systems.
PACT	: Prescribing Analysis and Cost.
	Pressure At Catheter`s Tip.(Ref. pressure measurement in expiratory phase).
PACTD	: Pulmonary Artery Catheter Thermodilution (Thermisters).(Ref. used on the ICU and during major surgery).
PACU	: Post-Anesthetic Care Unit. (USA).
PAD	: Peripheral Arterial Disease.
	Personally Administered Drug. (USA).
	Public Access Defibrillation.
PADSS	: Post-Anesthesia Discharge Scoring System. (USA).
PAE	: Possible Analgesic Effect.
PAEDS (Paed)	: Paediatrics.
PAF	: Performance Assessment Framework.

Platelet-Activating Factor.

Posterior Auricular Flap.

PAFC : Pulmonary Artery Flotation Catheter.

PAFSC : Pharmaceutical Affairs and Food Sanitation. (USA).

PAH : Para-Aminohippuric (Acid.)

PAI : Plasminogen Activator Inhibitor.

Propofol-Alfentanil Infusion.

PAIVMs : Passive Accesory Intervertebral Movements.

PAK : Pancreas after Kidney (Transplantation.)

PAL : Physical Activity Level.

Posterior Axillary Line.

PALS : Paediatric Advanced Life Support.

Patient Advice and Liaison Service.

Patient Advocacy and Liaison Service. (USA).

PAM : Post-Auricular Muscle.

Pofession Allied to Medicine.

PAN : Perinuclear Anti-Neutrophilic.

Polyarteritis Nodosa.

P-ANCA(p-ANCA): Perinuclear Anti-neutrophilic Cytoplasmic
Antibody.

PANDO : Primary Acquired Nasolacrimal Duct Obstruction.

PANSS : Positive and Negative Symptom Scale.

Positive and Negative Syndrome Scale.

PaO2 : Partial Pressure of Oxygen (in arterial blood).

PAOD : Peripheral Arterial Occlusive Disease.

PAOP : Pulmonary Artery Occlusion Pressure.

Pap : Papanicolaou`s Smear (or Stain Test).

PAP : Peak Airway Pressure.

Placental Alkaline Phosphatase.

Positive Airway Pressure.

Primary Atypical Pneumonia.

Prostatic Acid Phosphatase.

Pulmonary Artery Pressure.

PAPP-A : Pregnancy-Associated Plasma Protein A.

PAR : Perennial Allergic Rhinitis.

Physical Activity Ratio.

Post-Anaesthetic Recovery (Room).

PARAS : Postauricular and Retroauricular Scalping (Flap).

PARPs	: Pathogen Associated Recognition Patterns.
PAS	: Para-Aminosalicylic Acid.
	Patient Admission Service (Database).
	Periodic Acid-Schiff.
	Posterior Airway Space.
PASE	: Physical Activity Scale for Elderly.
PASM	: Pain and Substance Misuse.
PAT	: Pancreas Alone Transplantation.
	Paroxysmal Atrial Tachycardia.
	Peer Assessment Tool.
	Pulmonary Artery Hypertension.
P&T	: Pharmacy and Therapeutics (Committee). (USA).
PATE	: Prolonged Acute Tissue Expansion.
PAVA	: Pelargonic Acid Vanillylamide.
PAVMs	: Pulmonary Arterio-Venous Malformations.
Paw	: Airway Pressure.
PAWP	: Pulmonary Artery Wedge Pressure.
Pb	: Lead
PB	: Peripheral Blood.
	Placental Biopsy.
	Professional Body.
PBC	: Patient-Based Commissioning.
	Primary Biliary Chirrhosis.
PBF	: Pulmonary Blood Flow.
PBI	: Protein-Bound Iodine.
PBL	: Peripheral Blood Lymphocytes.
PBLI	: Practice-Based Learning and Improvement.
PBLS	: Paediatric Basic Life Support.
PBMs	: Pharmaceutical Benefit Managers. (USA).
PBMC	: Peripheral Blood Mononuclear Cell.
PbO$_2$	: Partial Pressure of Brain Oxygen.
PBPCs	: Peripheral Blood Progenitor Cells.
PbR	: Payment by Results. (Ref. payment to NHS hospitals by the **DoH**).
PBS	: Phosphate-buffered Saline.
	Peripheral Blood Smear.
PBSC	: Peripheral Blood Stem Cells.

PBSGL : Practice-Based Small Group Learning.(Ref. Learning method by General Practitioners).

PBZ : Phenylbutazone.

PC(p.c) : post cibum. (Ref. Latin for; "after food").

PCA : Patient-Controlled Analgesia.
Perchloracetic Acid. (Ref. in Neonatal hypoglycaemia testing).
Personal Care Attendant.

PCB : Post Coital Bleeding.

PCC : Post-coital Contraception.
Prothrombin Complex Concentrate. (Ref. used in Coagulation tests).

PCD : Primary Ciliary Dyskinesia.
Programmed Cell Death.

PCDS : Palliative Care Day Services.

PCE : Pericardial Effusion.
Pulmo-Cutaneous Exchange.

PCEA : Patient Controlled Epidural Analgesia.

PCEFs : Peak Cough Expiratory Flows.

PCF : Palliative Care Formulary.
Posterior Cranial Fossa.

PCG : Primary Care Group.

PCH : Paroxysmal Cold Haemoglobinuria.

PChE : Plasma Cholinesterase.

PCHR : Personal Child Health Record.

PCI : Percutaneous Coronary Intervention.

PCIA : Patient Controlled Interventions Analgesia.

PCIP : Primary Care Investment Plan.

PCKD : Polycystic Kidney Disease

PCL : Plasma Cell Leukaemia.
Posterior Cruciate Ligament.

PCM : Protein-Calorie Malnutrition.

PCMX : Parachlorometaxylenol

PCN(Pen.) : Penicillin.

PCN : Percutaneous Nephrostomy.

PCNA : Proliferating Cell Nuclear Antigen.

PCNL : Percutaneous Nephrolithotomy.

PCNSL : Primary Central Nervous System (**CNS**) Lymphoma.

PCO : Polycystic Ovaries.

Primary Care Organisation. (Formally **PCT**).

PCO2 (pCO2): Partial Pressure of Carbon Dioxide (in Blood).

PCOS : Polycystic Ovary Syndrome.

PCP : Pneumocystis Carinnii Pneumonia.

Phenycyclidine. (Ref. in Ketamine structure).

Primary Care Physician. (USA).

Primary Care Provider.

PcPAP : Periodic-controlled Positive Airway Pressure.

PCPS : Post-**CABG** Pain Syndrome.

PCR : Percutaneous Coronary Artery Revascularisation.

Phospho-Creatine.

Polymerase Chain Reaction. (Ref. Pulmonary vasoactive effects in Gancher Disease and with Sevoflurane use.)

Protein Catabolic Rate.

PCRA : Patient-Controlled Regional Analgesia.

PCS : Patient Controlled Sedation.

Post-concussion Syndrome.

Pulp Canal Sealer.

PCSS : Primary Care Support Services.

PCT : Patent Cooperation Treaty.

Porphyria Cutanae Tarda (or Porphyria Cutaneous Tarde).

Postcoital Test.

Primary Care Trust.

Procalcitonin. (Ref. levels of and patients outcome in **ICU**).

Prothrombin Clotting Time.

Proximal Convoluted Tubule.

PCTs : Primary Care Trusts.(Now Primary Care Organisations; **PCOs**).

PCTA : Percutaneous Transluminal Coronary Angioplasty.

PCV : Packed Cell Volume.

Pressure Controlled Ventilation.

PCWP : Pulmonary Capillary Wedge Pressure.

PD(PDis.)	: Parkinson`s Disease.
PD	: Panic Disorder.
	Peritoneal Dialysis.
	Personality Disorder.
	Pharmacodynamics.
	Pupillary Diameter. (Ref. in Ophthalmology).
PDA	: Patent Ductus Arteriosus.
PDB	: Paget`s Disease of Bone.
PDC	: Paediatric Diabetes Care.
PDD	: Parkinson`s Disease with Dementia.
	Passive Developmental Disorder.
	Pervasive Development Disorder.
	Premenstrual Dysphoric Disorder.
	Predicted Date of Discharge.
PDE 111	: Phosphodiesterase type 111.
PDF	: Portable Document Format.(Ref. e.g. as used in BMJ Research Files).
PDGF	: Platelet-derived Growth Factor.
PDGFR	: Platelet-derived Growth Factor Receptor.
PDH	: Past Dental History.
PDL	: Periodontal Ligament.
PDM	: Predentin Matrix.
PDMA	: Prescription Drug Marketing Act. (USA).
PDMS	: Polydimethylsiloxane.
PDNV	: Post-discharge Nausea and Vomiting.
PDP	: Personal Development Plan.
	Postnatal Depression Scale.
	Prescription Drug Plan. (USA).
PDPE	: Psychologically Determined Paroxysmal Events.
PDPH	: Post-Dural Puncture Headache.
PDS	: Pendred Syndrome.
	Polydioxanone Sutures.
PDT	: Percutaneous Dilatational Tracheostomy.
	Photodynamic Therapy.
PDUFA	: Prescription Drug User`s Fee Act. (USA).
PDUO	: Previous Day`s Urine Output.
PDW	: Platelet Distribution Width.

PE	: Pharyngoesophageal.
	Phenytoin Equivalent.
	Plasma Exchange.
	Pleural Effusion.
	Pulmonary Embolism.
PEA	: Persistent Electrical Activity.
	Pulseless Electrical Activity.
PEBP	: Prophylactic Epidural Blood Patch.
PEC	: Professional Executive Committee (of the **PCT**).
PEEP	: Positive End-Expiratory Pressure.
PEF	: Peak Expiratory Flow.
PEFR	: Peak Expiratory Flow Rate.
PEG	: Percutaneous Endoscopic Gastrostomy.
	Polyethylene Glycol.
PEI	: Pancreatic Exocrine Insufficiency.
PEIT	: Percutaneous Ethanol Injection Therapy.(Ref.
	management of Parathyroid Hyperplasia.)
PEJ	: Percutaneous Endoscopic Jejunostomy.
PELD	: Pediatric End-stage Liver Disease. (USA).
PEM	: Protein-Energy Malnutrition.
	Prescription Event Monitoring. (USA).
PEP	: Positive Expiratory Pressure.
	Post-Exposure Prophylaxis.
PEPAC	: Patient Pre-operative Assessment Clinic.
PERI	: Pharmaceutical Education and Research Institute. (USA).
PERLA	: Pupils Equal and Reactive to light and Accommodation.
PERT	: Pancreatic Enzyme Replacement Therapy.
PES	: Plastic Endosurgical System.
	Programmed Electrical Stimulation.
	Progress Evaluation Scale.
PESA	: Percutaneous Epididymal Sperm Aspiration.
PESS	: Powered Endoscopic Sinus Surgery.
PET	: Paediatric Tracheal Tube.
	Positron Emission Tomography.
	Pre-Eclampsia Toximia.
PEWS	: Paediatric Early Warning System Score.
PF	: Peak Flow.

	Platelet Function.
	Prothrombin Fragment.
PFA	: Platelet Function Analysis.
	Profunda Femoris Artery.
PFA–100	: Platelet Function Analyser (or Monitor).
PFAPA	: Periodic Fever and Pharyngitis and Cervical Adenitis(Syndrome).
PFAGH	: Penalty, Frustration, Anxiety, Guilt. Hostility.
PFC	: Persistent Foetal Circulation.
	Purified Fibrillar Collagen.
PFGE	: Pulse-field Gel Electrophoresis.
PFI	: Private Finance Initiative.
PFJ	: Patello-Femoral Joint.
PFK	: Phospho-Fructokinase.
PFO	: Patent Foramen Ovale.
PFPS	: Patello-Femoral Pain Syndrome.
PFR	: Peak Flow Rate.
PFSB	: Pharmaceutical and Food Safety Bureau. (USA).
PFTs	: Pulmonary Function Tests.
PG	: Prostaglandin.
PGA	: Patient Global Assessment. (Ref. in Pain control).
	Polyglycolic Acid.
PGADS	: Patient Global Assessment of Disease Status.
PGD	: Patient Group Directions. (Ref. Written directions relating to Supply and Administration of Prescriptions on-line).
	Pre-Implantation Genetic Diagnosis.
PGDF	: Platelet-derived Growth Factor.
PGDH	: Prostaglandin-degrading Enzyme 15-Hydroxyprostaglandin dehydrogenase.
PGE$_1$	: Prostaglandin E $_1$.
PGE$_2$	: Prostaglandin E $_2$.
PGI	: Peripheral Glyceral Injection.
PGI $_2$	: Prostaglandin I $_2$
PGL	: Persistent Generalised Lympadenopathy.
PGSR	: Psychogalvanic Skin Response.
PGSRA	: Psychogalvanic Skin Response Audiometry.

PGV	: Proximal Gastric Vagotomy.
pH	: Puissance d'Hydrogen (or Potential of Hydrogen).
PH	: Public Health.
PHA	: Polyhydroxy-Acid.
PHAs	: Polycyclic Aromatic Hydrocarbons.(Ref. to their adverse effects on Liver Cytochrome P450 enzymes.)
Pharm	: Pharmacy.
PHB	: Personal Health Budget.
PHBS	: Pseudo-Hypoxic Brain Swelling.
PHCHR	: Parent-Held Child Health Record.
PHCTs	: Primary Health Care Teams.
	Primary Health Care Trusts.
Ph.D	: Doctor of Philosophy.
p**he**	: Phenylalanine.
PHEC	: Pre-Hospital Emergency Care.
PHeL	: Public Health electronic Library.
p**Hi**	: Gastric Intramucosal **pH.** (Ref. Acidity).
PHI	: Primary Human Immuno-deficiency Virus (**HIV**) Infection.
PHLS	: Public Health Laboratory Service.
PHMC	: Public Health Medical Council (or Committee).
PHO	: Public Health Observatory.
PHOSC	: Public Health Overview and Security Committee.
PHP	: Practitioner Health Programme.(Ref. Healthcare programme by **BMA**).
	Primary Hyperparathyroidism.
	Pseudohypoparathroidism.
	Public Health Programme.
PHQ	: Patient Health Questionnaire.
PhRMA	: Pharmaceutical Reasearch and Manufacturers of America. (USA).
PHTC	: Pre-Hospital Trauma Course.
PHTN (PHT)	: Pulmonary Hypertension.
p**HVA**	: Plasma Homovanillic Acid.
PHVD	: Post-Haemorrhagic Ventricular Dilatation.
Phy.	: Pharyngitis.
	Physician.
Physio.	: Physiotherapy.

Physiol.	: Physiology.
PI	: Protease Inhibitor. (Ref. in treatment of **HIV**).
	Pulmonary (valve) Insufficiency (or Incompetence).
PIA	: Prolonged Infantile Apnoea.
PIAG	: Patient Information Advisory Group.
PIC	: Paediatric Intensive Care.
	Peripheral Indwelling Catheter.
PICC	: Peripherally Inserted Central Catheter.
PiCCO	: Pulse Contour Cardiac Output.
PICU	: Paediatric Intensive Care Unit.
PID	: Pelvic Inflammatory Disease.
	Position Indicating Device.
	Primary Immunodeficiency Disease.
	Prolapsed Intervertebral Disc.
PIE	: Plan, Intervention, Evaluation.
	Pulmonary Interstitial Emphysema.
PIENO-2000	: Parkinson's Information Exchange Network 2000. (USA).
PIFT	: Platelet Immunofluorescence Tests.
PIH	: Post Inflammatory Hyperpigmentation.
	Pregnancy-Induced Hypertension.
	Prolactin-Inhibiting Hormone.
PILs	: Patient Information Leaflets.
PIMs	: Paediatric Index of Mortality (Scores).
PIN	: Posterior Interosseous Nerve.
PIP	: Peak Inspiratory Pressure.
	Positive Inspiratory Pressure.
	Proximal Interphalangeal.
	Public Information Programme.
PIPE	: Pharmacologically Induced Penile Erection.
PIPJ	: Proximal Interphalangeal Joint.
PIPP	: Premature Infant Pain Profile.
PIS	: Poisons Information Services.
PIT	: Physician in Training.
PJC	: Porcelain Jacket Crown.

PJP	: Pneumocytis Jiroveci Pneumonia. (Ref. Pneumocytis Carinii Pneumonia)
PJRT	: Permanent Junctional Reciprocating Tachycardia.
PK	: Pharmacokinetics.
	Pyruvate Kinase.
PKC	: Protein Kinase.(Ref. inhibitory effect on Local Anaesthetics in post-operative Hyperalgesia).
PKD	: Polycystic Kidney Disease.
PKPD	: Pharmacokinetic-Pharmacodynamic (modelling).
PKR	: Photorefractive Keratotomy.
PKU	: Phenylketonuria.
PL	: Palmaris Longus.
	Perception of Light.
PLA	: Peri-Laryngeal Airway. (Ref. the Cobra **PLA**).
PLAB	: Professional and Linguistic Assessments Board.
PLE	: Protein-losing Enteropathy.
PLG	: Patients Liaison Group.
PLGA	: Polymorphous Low-Grade Adenocarcinoma.
PLI	: Professional Liability Insurance. (USA).
	Pulmonary Leak Index.
PLLA	: Poly-L-Lactic Acid.
PLM	: Pro-seal Laryngeal Mask Airway.
PLP	: Partial Laryngopharyngectomy.
	Phantom Limb Pain.
	Placenta Alkaline Phosphatase.
PLSVC	: Persistent Left Superior Vena Cava.(Ref. an anomalous Venous drainage).
Plts.	: Platelets.
PM	: Pectoralis Major.
	Polymyositis.
	Poor Metaboliser.
	Post-Mortem.
	Premolar.
PMA	: Post-Menstrual Age.
	Phorbol-Myristate Acetate.

PMB	: Post-Menopausal Bleeding.
PMC	: Pseudomembranous Colitis.
PMCA	: Plasmalemmal Calcium efflux.
PMCPA	: Prescription Medicines Code of Practice Authority.
PMD	: Post-Micturition Dribbling.
PMDA	: Pharmaceutical and Medical Devices Agency.
PMDD	: Premenstrual Dysphoric Disorder.
PMDI	: Propellant Metered Dose Inhaler.
PMETB	: Postgraduate Medical Education and Training Board.
PMF	: Progressive Massive Fibrosis.
PMFL	: Progressive Multifocal Leucoencephalopathy.
PMG	: Phonomyography. (Ref. used in monitoring neuro-muscular block).
PMH	: Paroxysmal Nocturnal Haemoglobinuria. Past Medical History. Previous Medical History.
PMI	: Point of Maximal Impulse. Post-operative Myocardial Infarction.
PML	: Progressive Multifocal Leukoencephalopathy. Promyelocytic Leukaemia.
PMLE	: Polymophous Light Eruption.
PMMA	: Polymethylmethacrylate.(Ref. Acrylic Bone Cement used in Orthopaedics).
PMN	: Polymorphonuclear Neutrophils.
PMNCs	: Polymorphonuclear Cells.
PMP	: Previous Menstrual Period.
PMR	: Percutaneous Myocardial Revascularisation. Polymyalgia Rheumatica.
PMRAFNS	: Princess Mary`s Royal Air Force Nursing Service.
PMS	: Personal Medical Service. Premenstrual Syndrome. Post-Marketing Surveillance. (USA).
PMT	: Parenchymal Marker Technique. Pre-Menstrual Tension. (see under **PMS**).
PMTs	: Pain Measurement Tools.
PMV	: Percutaneous Mitral Valvotomy.
PMVC	: Pulmonary Microvascular Cytology.

PN	: Parenteral Nutrition
	Postnasal.
	Postnatal.
	Practice Nurse.
	Pyelonephritis.
PNA	: Psychiatric Nurses Association.
PNB	: Peripheral Nerve Block.
PNC	: Postnatal Clinic.
PND	: Paroxysmal Nocturnal Dyspnoea.
	Postnatal Depression.
	Postnasal Drip.
PNET	: Primitive Neuroectodermal Tumour.
PNF	: Proprioneuro-facilitation.
PNH	: Paroxysmal Nocturnal Haemoglobinuria.
PNI	: Psycho-neuro-immunology.
PNS	: Peripheral Nerve Stimulator.
	Peripheral Nervous System. (USA).

PO	: Pulmonary Oedema.
PO(POp /Post op.): Post-operative.	
PO (po)	: Per os (or Per Oram or Orally).
PO$_2$ (pO$_2$)	: Partial pressure of Oxygen.
PO$_{4++}$	: Phosphate.
POA	: Power of Attorney.
POAG	: Primary Open Angle Glaucoma.
PoC	: Products of Conception.
POC	: Plan of Care.
	Point of Care.
	Pre-surgical Orthopaedic Correction.
POCD	: Post-Operative Cognitive Dysfunction (or Decline).
POCS	: Posterior Circulation Stroke.
POCT	: Point of Care Testing.
POCU	: Post-Operative Care Unit.
POFs	: Polymer Optic Fibres.
POG	: Progress in Obstetrics and Gynaecology.
POGO	: Percentage of Glottic Opening.
POISE	: Per-Operative Ischaemic Evaluation.(Ref. trial on mortality in patients on treatment with Beta-blockers).

POM	: Prescription-Only Medicines.
POMA	: (Tinetti) Performance Oriented Mobility Assessment.
POMC	: Pro-opiomelanocortin.
POMS	: Prescription Only Medicines.
	Profile of Mood States.
PNS	: Post-Nasal Space.
	Post-Nasal Spine (of the Hard Palate).
PONV	: Post-operative Nausea and Vomiting.
POP	: Plaster of Paris.
	Progestrone-Only Pill.
POPADAD	: Prevention of Progression of Arterial Disease and Diabetes.
PORC	: Post-Operative Residual Curarisation.
PORP	: Partial Ossicular Reconstruction Prothesis.
POS	: Point of Service.
post.	: Posterior.
POTS	: Postural Orthostatic Tachycardia Syndrome.
POU	: Point of Use.
POVA	: Protection of Vulnerable Adults.
POVL	: Post-Operative Visual Loss.
PP	: Placenta Previa.
	Precocious Puberty.
	Private Patient.
PPA	: Parapharyngeal Abscess.
	Prescription Pricing Authority.
PPAM	: Pneumatic Post-Amputation Mobility.
PPAR	: Peroxisome Proliferator—Activated Receptors. (Ref. receptor for **UGT**).
PPD	: Personal and Professional Development.
	Progressive Perceptive Deafness.
	Purified Protein Derivative.
PPE	: Personal Protective Equipment.
PPF	: Plasma Protein Fraction.
	Priorities and Planning Framework
PPG	: Post-prandial Glucose.
PPH	: Post-Partum Haemorrhage.
	Primary Pulmonary Hypertension.

PPHN	: Persistent Pulmonary Hypertension of the Newborn.
PPI	: Patient and Public Involvement.
	Private Patients Income.
	Proton Pump Inhibitor.
PPM	: Permanent Pacemaker.
ppm	: Parts per million.
PPN	: Peripheral Parenteral Nutrition.
PPOs	: Preferred Provider Organizations. (USA).
PPP	: Personal Professional Profile.
PPPE	: Prolonged Postpeel Erythema.
PPROM	: Preterm Prelabour Rupture of Membranes.
	Preterm Prolonged Rupture of Membranes.
PPRS	: Pharmaceutical Price Regulation Scheme.
PPS	: Parapharyngeal Space.
	Plasma Protein Solution.
	Prospective Payment System (for Nursing facilities). (USA).
PPT	: Pressure Pain Threshold.
PPTA	: Plasma Protein Therapeutics Association. (USA).
PPTL	: Pressure Pain Tolerance Level.
PPV	: Positive Pressure Ventilation.
PPVs	: Positive Predictive Values.(Ref. e.g. the likelihood of Ovarian Cancer).
PR	: Per Rectum.
	Prostate. (USA).
	Prothrombin Ratio.
PRA	: Plasma Renin Activity.
PRCA	: Pure Red Cell Aplasia.
PRCP	: President of the Royal College of Physicians.
PRD	: Pupillary Reflex Dilatation.
Prem	: Premature.
Pre-op	: Pre-operative.
PREP	: Post-Registration Education and Practice (Standards).
PRES	: Posterior Reversible Encephalopathy Syndrome.(Ref. hypertensive crisises).
PRG	: Percutaneous Radiological Gastrostomy.
PRH	: Prolactin-Releasing Hormone.

PRHO   : Pre-Registration House Officer.
PrI   : Prolactin.
PRI   : Propofol-Remifentanil Infusion. (Ref. in General
                   Anaesthesia).
PRICE   : Protection, Rest, Ice, Compression, Elevation.
PRINCE   : Projects In Controlled Environment.
PRIS   : Propofol Infusion Syndrome.
PRISMA   : Prevention and Recovery Information System for
                   Monitoring Analysis.
PRL (PrL or PL): Prolactin.
PRMP   : Pharmion Risk Management Programme.
PRN (prn)   : Pro re nata. (Ref. Latin for; as required/whenever
                   required or necessary).
PROACT   : Prolyse in Acute Cerebral Thromboembolism.
Prof.   : Professor.
PROM   : Passive Range of Motion.
                   Patient-reported Outcome Measure.
                   Pre-labour (Premature) Rupture of the Membranes..
                   Prolonged Rupture of Membranes. (Ref. in Obstetrics).
PROMESS   : Programme on Essential Medicines and Supplies.
PrP   : Prion Protein.
PRR   : Preventive Resin Restoration.
PRT   : Proton Radiation Therapy.
PRV   : Polycythemia rubra vera.

PS   : Per Speculum.
                   Pressure Support.
                   Psoas muscle. (USA).
                   Pulmonary Stenosis.
P/S   : Presenting Symptoms.
Psa   : Psoriatic Arthritis.
                   Pacing System Analyser.
PSA   : Prostate Specific Antigen.
PSARP   : Posterior Sagittal Anorectoplasty.
PSB   : Bronchoscopic Specimen Brushing.
PSC   : Posterior Semicircular Canal.
                   Primary Sclerosing Cholangitis.
PSCC   : Posterior Semi-circular Canal.

PSCT	: Pain and Symptom Control Team.
PSD	: Patient Specific Direction. (USA).
	Pneumosinus Dilatans.
PSE	: Present State Examination.
	Portal Systemic Encephalopathy.
PSEF	: Plastic Surgery Educational Foundation.
PSF	: Posterior Spinal Fusion.
PSH	: Past Surgical History.
PSHE	: Personal, Social, and Health Education.
PSI	: Paediatric Speech Intelligibility (Test).
	Patient Safety Index.
	Pneumonia Severity Index.
PSIS	: Posterior Superior Iliac Spine.
PSM	: Pan-systolic Murmur.
PSNI	: Perceived Support Network Inventory.
PSNL	: Partial Sciatica Nerve Ligation. (Ref. pain score in mice test).
PSNP	: Progressive Supranuclear Palsy.
PSP	: Phenolsulfonphalein.
PSS	: Physiological Scoring System.
PST	: Promontory Stimulation Test.
PSTTs	: Placenta Site Trophoblast Tumours.
PSURs	: Periodic Safety Update Reports. (USA).
PSV	: Pressure Support Ventilation.
	Primary Systemic Vasculitis.
Psyc.	: Psychology.
PSYCH	: Psychiatry.
PSYM	: Parasympathetic.
PT	: Permeability Tension.
	Physiotherapist.
	Prothrombin Time.
	Pulmonary Tuberculosis. (see under **PTB**).
PTA	: Pancreas Transplant Alone.
	Peritonsillar Abscess.
	Post-Traumatic Amnesia.
	Prior to Admission.
PTB	: Patellar Tendon Bearing.

Pulmonary Tubercle Bacillus (Pulmonary Tuberculosis).

PTC : Percutaneous Transhepatic Cholengiopancreatography.
Percutaneous Transhepatic Cholengiogram.

PTCA : Percutaneous Transluninal Coronary Angiography (or Angioplasty).

PTE : Pulmonary Thromboembolism.

PTFE : Polytetrafluoroethylene(graft).(Ref. used in bypass for superior vena cava).

PT-Fg : Prothrombin Time-derived Fibrinogen.

PTFL : Posterior Talofibular Ligament.

PTH : Parathyroid Hormone.

PTL : Pre-Term (Premature) Labour.

PTLD : Post-Transplant Lymphoproliferative Disorder.

PTP : Physical Work-pressure Product.(Ref. mechanical load of humidifying Devices).

PTR : ProthrombinRatio.

PTS : Permanent Threshold Shift.
Post-Thrombotic Syndrome.

PTSD : Post-Traumatic Stress Disorder.

PTT : Pulse Transit Time.(Ref. Pulse beat-to-beat cardiovascular information; e.g. in pregnancy induced hypertension. **PIH**).
Partial Thromboplastin Time.

PTTK : Partial Thromboplastin Time with Kaolin.

PTU : Propylthiouracil.

PTV : Patient-Triggered Ventilation.

PU : Pass (or Passed) Urine.
Peptic Ulcer.
Prescribing Unit.

PUBS : Percutaneous Umbilical Blood Sampling.

PUD : Peptic Ulcer Disease.

PUFA : Polyunsaturated Fatty Acids.

PUJ : Pelvis-ureteric Junction.

PUL : Pregnancy of Unknown Location.

PUO : Pyrexia of Unknown Origin.

PUPP : Pruritic Urticarial Papules and Placques of Pregnancy.

PUS : Prostate Ultrasound.

PUSH   : Pressure Ulcer Scale for Healing.

PUV   : Posterior Urethral Valve.

PUVA   : Psoralen plus Ultraviolet A(Waves). (Ref. previously used as photochemotherapy treatment for Psoriasis but now discontinued).

PUVB   : Psoralen plus Ultraviolet B (Light).

PV   : Peak Velocity.
Pemphigus Vulgaris.
Per Vagina.
Plasma Viscosity.
Plasma Volume.
Pressure Volume.
Pulmonary Valve.

PVA   : Partial Villous Atrophy.
Polyvinyl Alcohol. (Ref. used in embolising tumours).

PVARP   : Post-Ventricular Atrial Refractory Period.

PVB   : Paravertebral Block.
Premature Ventricular Beat.

PVC   : Parked Volume (Red) Cells.
Polyvinyl Chloride.
Premature Ventricular Contraction.

PVD   : Peripheral Vascular Disease.
Peripheral Vestibular Deficit.

PVE   : Prosthetic Valve Endocarditis.

PVFD   : Paradoxical Vocal Fold Dysfunction.

PVH   : Periventricular Haemorrhage.

PVL   : Panton-Valentine Leukocidin.(Ref. a Cytotoxin produced by 2% of Staphalococcus aureaus bacteria).
Periventricular Leucomalacia.

PVNS   : Pigmented Villonodular Tenovagosynovitis.

PVOD   : Peripheral Vascular Occlusive Disease.

PVP   : Pulmonary Venous Pressure..

PVR   : Pulmonary Vascular Resistance.

PVRI   : Pulmonary Vascular Resistance Index.

PVT   : Paroxysmal Ventricular Tachycardia.
Polymorphic Ventricular Tachycardia.

PWA	: Platelet Works Analyser.
PWI	: Perfusion Weighted Imaging.
PWS	: Prader-Willi Syndrome.
Px	: Prescription (or Prescribe).
PXE	: Pseudoxanthoma Elastine.
PXR	: Pregnane-X Receptor.
PYY	: Peptide YY. (Ref. an appetite control hormone found in the lower Gut).
PZ	: Pancreozymin.
PZA	: Pyrazinamide.
PZD	: Partial Zona Dissection.
PZI	: Protamine Zinc Insulin.
Q	: Cardiac Output.
QA	: Quality Assurance.
QALY	: Quality Adjusted Life Years.(Ref. in relation to vaccination protection).
QARANC	: Queen Alexandra`s Royal Army Nursing Corps.
QARNNS	: Queen Alexandra`s Royal Naval Nursing Service.
Qd	: Every day.
Qds (qds)	: Quater die sumendum. (Ref. Latin for; "to be taken four times daily").
QEEG	: Quantitative analysis of the Electroencephalogram.
QF	: Qualifying Factor.
QF-PCR	: Quantitative Fluorescent Polymerase Chain Reaction.
Qh	: Every hour.
QI	: Quality Improvement.
QID(Qid or qid)	: Quarter in die. (Latin for;" Four times a day").
QIDN	: Queen`s Institute of District Nursing.
QIPP	: Quality, Innovation, Productivity and Prevention.

QLS	: Quality of Life Scale.
QMAS	: Quality Management and Analysis System.
QN	: Qualified Nurse.
QNI	: Queen's Nursing Institute.
Qod	: Every other day.
QOF	: Quality and Outcomes Framework.
QoL	: Quality of Life.
QPs	: Qualified Persons.
QPP	: Quality from Patients Perspective.
qqh	: Quata quaque hora. (Ref. Latin for; "every four hours").
QRH	: Quick Reference Handbook (Medical).
QSART	: Quantitative Sudomotor Axon Reflex Tests.
QUART	: Quadrantectomy, Axillary Dissection,Radiotherapy.
QUID	: Quantitative Ingredient Declaration.
QUO	: Quality of Reporting of Meta-analysis.
Qw-MI	: Q-wave Myocardial Infarction, **MI**.
R	: Respiration.
	Rib.
	Right.
RA	: Refractory Anaemia.
	Retinoic Acid.
	Retrograde Amnesia.
	Rheumatoid Arthritis.
	Right-Atrium.
RAA	: Renin-Angiotensin-Aldosterone System.
RAAA	: Rupture of Abdominal Aortic Aneurysm.
RAAS	: Renin-Angiotensin-Aldosterone System.
RACE	: Rate Control versus Electrical Cardioversion.

RAD : Right Axis Deviation.
RADAR : Royal Association for Disability and Rehabilitation.
RADS : Reactive Airway Dysfunction Syndrome.
RAE : Ring-Adair-Elwyn. (Ref. an Endotracheal Tube used in Anaesthesia).
RAFF : Rectus Abdominis Free Flap.
RAH : Right Atrial Hypertrophy.
RAI : Rheumatoid Attitude Index.
Radioactive Iodine.
RAIU : Radioactive Iodine Uptake.
RAFEA : Radio Frequency Endometrial Ablation.
RAM : Rectus Abdominis Musculocutaneous (Flap).
RAMCF : Rectus Abdominis Myocutaneous Flap.
RANK : Receptor Activator of Nuclear Kappa B.
RANKL : Receptor Activator of Nuclear Kappa B Ligand.
RAO : Right Anterior Oblique (Angiocardiogram).
RAP : Right Atrial Pressure.
RAPA : Rheumatoid Particle Agglutination (Test).
rAPC : Recombinant Activated Protein C.
RAPD : Random Amplification of Polymorphic **DNA.**
RAS : Renin Angiotensin System.
Renal Artery Stenosis.
Reticular Activating System.
RASE : Rheumatoid Arthritis Self-Efficacy Scale.
RASJ : Radio-Immunoassay Techniques.
RAST : Radio-Allergosorbent Test. (Ref. Latex allergy testing).
RAT : Regional Action Team.
RATE : Regulatory Authority for Tissues and Embryos.
RAWP : Resource Allocation Working Party.

RBBB : Right Branch Bundle Block.
RBCs : Red Blood Cells.
RBE : Radio-Biological Effectiveness.
RBG : Random Blood Glucose.
RBI : Relative Benefit Increase.
Retinoblastoma gene.
RBS : Random Blood Sugar.
RBW : Real Body Weight.

RCA : Right Coronary Artery.
Royal College of Anaesthetists.
RCBF (rCBF): Regional Cerebral Blood Floor.
RCC : Recovery Care Center. (USA).
Red Cell Concentrate.
Red Cell Count.
Renal Cell Carcinoma.
RCGP : Royal College of General Practitioners.
RCM : Red Blood Cell Mass.
Royal College of Midwives.
RCN (Rcn) : Royal College of Nursing.
RCNT : Registered Clinical Nurse Teacher.
RCoA (RCA) : Royal College of Anaesthetists.
RCOG : Royal College of Obstetricians and Gynaecologists.
RCOphth. : Royal College of Ophthalmology.
RCP : Retruded Contact Position.
Royal College of Physicians.
RCPCH : Royal College of Paediatrics and Child Health.
RCPE : Royal College of Physicians of Edinburgh.
RCPSG : Royal College of Physicians and Surgeons of Glasgow.
RCR : Royal College of Radiologists.
RCRI : Revised Cardiac Risk Index.
RCS : Royal College of Surgeons.
RCSE : Royal College of Surgeons of Edinburgh.
RCT : Randomised Clinical Trial.
Root Canal Treatment.

RD : Registered Dietitian.
Risk Difference.
RDis. : Refsum`s Disease.
RDA : Recommended Daily Amount.
Recommended Dietary Allowance.
RDEB : Recessive Dystrophic Epidermolysis Bullosa.
RDH : Registered Dental Hygienist.
RDI : Recommended Dietary Intake.
Recommended Daily Intake.
Respiratory Distress Index.

rDNA	: Recombinant Deoxyribonucleic Acid.
RDS	: Rapidly Digestible Starch.
	Respiratory Distress Syndrome.
RDTs	: Rapid Diagnostic Tests.
RDW	: Red Blood Cell Distribution Width.
RE	: Response Entropy. (Ref. used in assessing nociception).
	Reticuloendothelium (or Reticuloendothelial).
	Right Eye.
ReA	: Reactive Arthritis.
REACH	: Reduction of Artherothrombosis for Continued Health.
REACT	: Rescue Angioplasty versus Conservative Therapy (Study).
REAIM	: Reach,Efficacy,Adoption, Impact, Maintenance.(Ref. programme network)
RECORD	: Rosiglitazone Evaluated for Cardiovascular Outcomes.
REE	: Resting Energy Expenditure.
REHAB	: Rehabilitation Evaluation of Hall and Baker.
REM	: Rapid Eye Movement.
REMS	: Rapid Emergency Medicine Score.
	Regional Examination of the Musculoskeletal System.
RES	: Reynold`s Empathy Scale.
RET	: Rational Emotive Therapy.
Retics.	: Reticulocytes.
RF	: Radio Frequency.
	Renal Failure.
	Rheumatic Fever.
	Rheumatoid Factor.
RFA	: Radiofrequency Ablation.
RFFF	: Radia Forearm Free Flap.
RFI	: Request for Information.
RFID	: Radiofrequency Identification Device.(Ref. chip with essential Data in form of Electronic Product Code: **EPC**).
RFLP	: Restriction Fragment Length Polymorphisms.
RFN	: Registered Fever Nurse. (USA).
RFPs	: Requests for Proposals. (USA).
RFT	: Respiratory Function Tests.

RGN : Registered General Nurse.

RH : Right Hypochondriac (of the Abdomen).
Rh : Rhesus (Factor).
Rheumatism.
RHA : Regional Health Authority.
Rh(D) : Rhesus D (Antigen).
RHD : Rhesus Haemolytic Disease.
Rheumatic Heart Disease.
RhF : Rheumatoid Factor.
RHV : Registered Health Visitor.

RI : Right Inguinal.
R-wave Interval. (Ref. on the **ECG**).
RIA : Radioimmunoassay.
RIBA : Radio-Immuno-Blot Assay. (USA).
RICES : Rest, Ice, Compression, Elevation,Splintting.
RIDDOR : Reporting Injuries, Diseases and Dangerous Occurrences
Regulations.
RIE : Recorded in Error.
RIF : Right Iliac Fossa.
RIG : Radiologically Inserted Gastrostomy.
RIMA : Reversible Inhibitor of Monoamine Oxidase (**MAO**).
Right Internal Mammary Artery.
RIMOA : Reversible Inhibitor of Monoamine Oxidase-A.
RIND : Reversible Ischaemic Neurologic Deficit.
rINN : Recommended International Non-proprietary Name.
RIOTT : Randomised Injectable Opiate Treatment Trial.
RIP : Respiratory Inductance Pneumography.
RIPA : Ristocetin-Induced Platelet Aggregation.

RK : Radial Keratotomy.
Right Kidney.
RLL : Right Lower Lobe.
RLMT : Resident Labour Market Test.
RLN : Recurrent Laryngeal Nerve.
RLNP : Recurrent Laryngeal Nerve Palsy.

RLQ   : Right Lower Quadrant (of the Abdomen).
RLS   : Restless Lgs Syndrome.

RM   : Recurring Miscarriage.
               Rectus (Abdominis) Muscle.
               Registered Midwife.
r m   : Rigor mortis.
RMHP   : Reserves Mental Health Programme.
RML   : Right Middle Lobe.
RMN   : Registered Mental Nurse. (Ref. see Psychiatric Nurse).
RMO   : Resident Medical Officer.
               Responsible Medical Officer.
RMP   : Risk Management Program. (USA).
RMR   : Resting Metabolic Rate.
RMS   : Rhabdomyosarcoma.
RMSE   : Root Mean Square Error.
RMSF   : Rocky Mountain Spotted Fever.
RMZ   : Right Middle Zone.

RN   : Registered Nurse.
RNA   : Ribonucleic Acid.
RNCC   : Registered Nursing Care Contributions.
RND   : Radical Neck Dissection.
RNI   : Reference Nutrient Intake.
RNIB   : Royal National Institute for the Blind.
RNMH   : Registered Nurse for the Mentally Handicapped.(Ref. for
               people with Learning Difficulties).
RNP   : Ribonucleoprotein.
RNPFN   : Royal National Pension Fund for Nurses.
RNS   : Rheumatology Nurse Specialist.
RNT   : Registered Nurse Tutor.
RNV   : Radio-Nuclide Ventriculography.

ROs   : Responsible Officers. (Ref. doctors who sign off
               recommendations for Revalidation).
ROA   : Right Occipito-Anterior.
ROAM   : Range of Active Movement.

ROC	: Receiver Operating Characteristic Curve.(Ref. the discrimination ability of Diagnostic different scores.)
RODAC	: Replicate Organism Detection and Counting.
ROM	: Range of Movement (or Motion).
ROOF	: Retro-Orbicularis Oculi Fat.
ROP	: Retinopathy of Prematurity.
	Right Occipito-Posterior.
ROS	: Reactive Oxygen Species. (Ref. in tissue damage and in infarction).
	Removal of Sutures.
	Review of Systems.
ROSC	: Return of spontaneous Circulation.
ROTEM	: Rotation Thromboelastography.(Ref. tests for Hyperfibrinolysis in **USA**).
RP	: Retinitis Pigmentosa.
RPA	: Recurrent Pleomorphic Adenoma.
	Recurrent-Pharyngeal Abscess.
RPC	: Right Pleural Cavity.
RPE	: Retinal Pigmented Epithelial (Cells or Layer).
RPGN	: Rapidly Progressive Glomerulonephritis.
RPLND	: Retroperitoneal Lymph-node Dissection.
RPLS	: Reversible Posterior Leukoencephalopathy Syndrome.
RPR	: Rapid Plasma Reagin. (A test for Syphilis).
RPS	: Radiation Protection Supervisor.
RPSGB	: Royal Pharmaceutical Society of Great Britain.
Rpt.	: Repeat.
	Report.
RQ	: Respiratory Quotient.
RR	: Recovery Room.
	Regain (Eye) Reflex.
	Relative Risk.
	Relative Ratio.
	Respiratory Rate.
RRI	: Relative Risk Increase.
RRIV	: R-R Interval Variability (on the **ECG**).

RRP : Recurrent Respiratory Papilloma (or Papillomatosis).
RRR : Rapid Response Report. (Ref. National Patients Safety Agency; **NPSA**).
Relative Risk Reduction.

RRT : Rapid Response Team.
Renal Replacement Therapy.
RRV : Right Renal Vein.

RS : Re-feeding Syndrome.
Resistant Starch.
Respiratory System.
RSA : Respiratory Sinus Arrhythmia.
RSBD : Rapid Eye Movement (**REM**) Sleep Behaviour Disorder.
RSD : Reflex Sympathetic Dystrophy.
Residual Standard Deviation.
RSH : Reproductive and Sexual Health.
RSI : Rapid Sequence Induction.
Repetitive Strain Injury.
RSIVI : Rapid Sequence Intravenous Induction.(Ref. inducing General Anaesthesia).
RSM : Royal Society of Medicine.
RSO : Resting Sweat Output.
RSS : Rotatory Sublaxation of Scaphoid.
RSV : Respiratory Syncytial Virus.

RT : Radiotherapy.
Rapid Tranquillization.
Reinforced Tube.(Ref. reinforced Endo-Tracheal Tube for Anaesthetic use).
Reverse Transcriptase.
Reverse Trendelenburg (position).
RTA : Renal Tubular Acidosis.
Road Traffic Accident.
Ruptured Tendon Archilles.
RTI : Respiratory Tract Infection.
rTPA : Recombinant Thrombin Plasminogen Activator.
RTP : Return to Practice.

RT-PCR	: Reverse Transcriptase-Polymerate Chain Reaction.
RTS	: Revised Trauma Score.
RUA	: Right Upper Arm.
RUCAM	: Roussel Uclaf Casuality Assessment Method.
RUL	: Right Upper Lobe.
RUQ	: Right Upper Quadrant (of the Abdomen).
RUR	: Really Useful Robots.
	Rossum`s Universal Robots.
RUTH	: Raloxifene Use for The Heart (Trial).
RUZ	: Right Upper Zone.
RV	: Residual Volume.
	Right Ventricle.
RVA	: Right Visual Acuity.
RVED	: Right Ventricle End-Diastolic (Area).
RVEDP	: Right Ventricular End-Diastolic Pressure.
RVESA	: Right Ventricle End-Systolic Area.
RVF	: Right Ventricular Function (or Failure).
RVH	: Right Ventricular Hypertrophy.
RVOT	: Right Ventricular Outflow Tract.
RVSW(I)	: Right Ventricular Stroke Work (Index).
RWMMAs	: Regional Wall Motion Abnormalities. (Ref. Ventricular wall movements in Systole).
Rx	: Treat or Treatment. (Ref. a Prescription sign).
Rxn	: Reaction.
RYGB	: Roux-en-Y Gastric Bypass.
RYRI	: Ryanodine Receptor Gene. (Ref. in Malignant Hyperpyrexia: **MH**).
s	: Second.
S	: Sacral.
	Schedule.
	Serum.
S 1–5	: Sacro-Spinal Segments 1-5.

SA	: Sino-Atrial.
	Sinuatrial (nodal branch of the Right Coronary Artery). (USA).
	Stable Anaesthesia.
S/A	: Suicide Attempt.
SAA	: Serum Amyloid-A (Ref. a protein related to acute inflammatory response).
	Serum Anticholinergic Activity.
SAC	: Safety Assessment Code. (Ref. likelihood of error and its effect on the patient).
	Scientific Advisory Committee.
	Special Advisory Committee (in Otolaryngology).
SACD	: Subacute Combined Degeneration of the Spinal Cord.
SACMILL	: Scientific Advisory Committee on Medical Implications of Less-Lethal (Weapons).
SACN	: Scientific Advisory Committee on Nutrition.
SACT	: Sino-Atrial Conduction Time.
SAD	: Seasonal Affective Disorder.
	Separation Anxiety Disorder.
	Social Anxiety and Distress (Scale).
SADs	: Supraglottic Airway Devices.
SADQ	: Severity of Alcohol Dependence Questionnaire.
SAE	: Sepsis Associated Encephalopathy.
SAECG	: Signal-Averaged **ECG.**
SAFE	: Saline versus Albumin in Fluid Evaluation.
SAG-M	: Saline Adenine Glucose-Mannitol.
SAH	: Subarachnoid Haemorrhage.
SAHSU	: Small Area Health Statistics Utilisation (Database).
SAID	: Specific Adaptations to Imposed Demand.
SALT	: Speech and Language Therapy (or Therapist).
SAM	: Systolic Anterior Motion (or Movement).
SAMBA	: Simulataneous Areolar Mastopexy and Breast Augmentation.
	Society for Ambulatory Anesthesia. (USA).
SA(N)	: Sinoatrial Node.
SANDS	: Stilbirth and Neonatal Death Society.
SaO2	: Arterial Oxygen Saturation.
SAP	: Single Assessment Process.

Systolic Arterial Pressure.

SAPS	: Simplified Acute Physiology Scores.
SAPV	: Systolic Arterial Pressure Variability.
SAQ	: Safety Attitudes Questionnaire
	Short Answer Question (Examination).
SAR	: Seasonal Allergic Rhinitis.
SARA	: Sexually-Acquired Reactive Arthropathy (or Arthritis).
SARI	: Serotonin Antagonist and Re-uptake Inhibitor.
SARS	: Severe Acute Respiratory Syndrome.
SAS	: Scottish Ambulance Service.
	Sedation-Agitation Scale.
	Self-rating Anxiety Scale.
	Staff and Associate Specialist.
	Sulfasalazine.
SASC	: Staff and Associate Specialist Committee.
SASM	: Scottish Audit of Surgical Mortality.
SASQ	: Single Alcohol Screening Questionnaire.
SAT	: Serum Aspartate Transferase.
SAWG	: Scientific Advice Working Group. (USA).
SB	: Spinal Bifida.
	Spontaneous Breathing.
	Stillbirth (or Stillborn).
S/B	: Seen by.
SBAR	: Situation, Background, Assessment and Response.
SBCU	: Special Baby Care Unit. (see under **SCBU**).
SBE	: Subacute Bactarial Endocarditis.
SBFT	: Small Bowel Follow-through (X-Ray).
SBN$_2$	: Single-Breath (expired) Nitrogen (slope).
SBO	: Small Bowel Obstruction.
SBP	: Spontaneous Bacterial Peritonitis.
	Systolic Blood Pressure.
SBR	: Serum Bilirubin.
	Spontaneous Baroreflex.
SBS	: Short Bowel Syndrome.
SBT	: Single Breath Test.
Sc	: Sigmoid Colon.

SC (s/c; sc)	: Subcutaneous.
SC	: Skin Conductance.
	Spinal Cord.
	Sterno-Clavicular (Joint).
	Sugar-coated.
SCA	: Sickle Cell Anaemia.
SCAN	: Schedules for Clinical Assessment in Neuropsychiatry.
SCAP	: Severe Community Acquired Pneumonia.
SCAT	: Standardised Concussion Assessment Tool.
SCATA	: Society for Computing And Technology in Anaesthesia.
SCBU	: Special Care Baby Unit.
SCC	: Squamous Cell Carcinoma.
SCCHN	: Squamous Cell Cancer of the Head and Neck.
SCCOT	: Standard Care versus Celecoxib Outcome Trial.
SCD	: Sequential-Pneumatic Compression Device.
	Sickle Cell Disease.
	Sudden Cardiac Death.
SCF	: Scientific Committee for Food (European).
	Stem Cell Factor.
SCFA	: Short Chain Fatty Acids.
SCFE	: Slipped Capital Femoral Epiphysis.
SCG	: Sodium Chromoglycate.
ScHARR	: Sheffield School of Health and Related Research.
Sci.	: Science.
SCI	: Spinal Cord Injury.
SCIA	: Superficial Circumflex Iliac Artery.
SCID	: Severe Combined Immunodeficiency.
SCJ	: Squamo-Columnar Junction. (Ref. Ecto-Endocervical junction).
SCL	: Subcortical Leucomalacia.
SCLE	: Sub-acute Cutaneous Lupus Erythematosus.
SCM	: Sterno-Cleiroido-Mastoid Muscle. (USA).
	Synovial Chondromatosis.
SCMT	: Sterno-Cleiroido-Mastoid Tumour.
SCNT	: Somatic Cell Nuclear Transfer.
SCODA	: Standing Conference on Drug Abuse.
SCORTEN	: Severity of Illness Score for Toxic Epidermal Necrolysis.

SCOUT	: Sibutramine Cardiovascular Outcomes Trial.(Ref. increased morbidity to Cardiovascular Disease by this Anti-Obesity drug: **now withdrawn**).
SCPHN	: Specialist Community Public Health Nurse.
SCr	: Serum Creatinine.
SCR	: Summary Care Record.
SCS	: Spinal Cord Stimulation.
SCT	: Sacrococcygeal Teratomas.
	Social Cognitive Therapy.
SCU	: Special Care Unit.
SCV	: Sub-Clavian Vein.
ScvO2	: Central venous Oxygen saturation.
SD(sd)	: Standard Deviation (Ref. in Statistics).
SD	: Single Dose.
	Spasmodic Dysphonia.
	Stroke Distance.
SDC	: Salivary Duct Carcinoma.
SDD	: Selective Decontamination of Digestive (Tract).
SDH	: Subdural Haematoma.
SDQ	: Strength and Difficulties Questionnaire.
SDS	: Slowly Digestible Starch.
	Sodium Dodecyl Sulphate.
	Symptom Distress Score.
SDSU	: Same-Day Surgical Unit.
se (s/e)	: Standard Error (Ref. in Statistics).
Se	: Selenium.
SE	: Self-efficacy.
	Side Effect.
	Standard Error.
	State Entropy. (Ref. in the assessment of nociception).
	Status Epilepticus.
SEA	: Significant Event Audit.
SEF	: Spectral Edge Frequency.
SEH	: Sub-Ependymal Haemorrhage.
SEHD	: Scottish Executive Health Department.
SELI	: Specific Expressive Language Impairment.
SEM	: Sports and Exercise Medicine.

	Standard Error of the Mean.
SEN	: Special Education Need.
	State Enrolled Nurse.
SENCO	: Special Education Needs Coordinator.
SEND	: Sub-Endothelial Deposit.
SENIC	: Study of efficacy of Nasocomial Infection Control (Project).
SEP	: Somatosensory Evoked Potential
	Systolic Ejection Period.
SEPD	: Sub-Epithelial Deposit.
SERMs	: Selective Oestrogen Receptor Modulators.
SESAM	: Society in Europe for Simulation Applied to Medicine.
SETFS	: South East Thames Foundation School.

SF	: Saphenofemoral.
SFA	: Saturated Fatty Acid.
	Superficial Femoral Artery.
SFD	: Small for Dates.
SFH	: Symphyseal-Fundal Height.
SFGA	: Small-for-Gestational Age.
SFJ	: Saphenofemoral Junction.
SFN	: Scalp,Finger Needle (Technique) : (Ref. difficult Airway management).

SG	: Specific Gravity.
SGA	: Small for Gestational Age.
SGB	: Stellate Ganglion Block.
SGC	: Salivary Gland Carcinoma.
SGE	: Second Gas Effect.(Ref. Nitrous Oxide Gas exchange in Anaesthesia).
SGH	: Sebaceous Gland Hyperplasia.
SGMI	: Silicon-filled Mammary Implant.
SGOT	: Serum Glutamic Oxaloacetic Transaminase;(now obsolete; see **SAT**)
SGPT	: Serum Glutamic-Pyruvic Transaminase (Activity).
SGS	: Sub-Glottic Stenosis.

| **SH** | : Self Harm. |

Social History.
Standard Heparin.

SHAs	: Strategic Health Authorities.
SHARE	: Scottish Health Authorities Revenue Equalisation.
SHARP	: Study of Heart and Renal Protection.
SHBG	: Sex-Hormone-Binding Globulin.
SHDU	: Surgical High Dependency Unit.
SHERP	: Systemic Human Error Reduction and Prediction (Approach).
SHFJV	: Superimposed High Frequency Jet Ventilation.
SHHD	: Scottish Home and Health Department.
SHIF	: Social Health Insurance Fund.
SHIP	: Self-Help in Pain (Groups).
SHL	: Sudden Hearing Loss.
SHO	: Senior House Officer.(Now obsolete in the U.K).
SHOT	: Serious Hazards of Transfusion.
SHOW	: Scottish Health on the Web.
SHRs	: Standardised Hospitalisation Ratios.
SHS	: Scientific Hospital Supplies.

SI	: Sacro-iliac.
	Soluble Insulin.
	Statutory Instrument.
SIADH	: Syndrome of Inappropriate Anti-diuretic Hormone (secretion).
SID	: Strong Ion Difference. (Ref. Normal Saline solution and Metabolic Acidosis).
SIDS	: Sudden Infant Death Syndrome.
SIE	: Stroke in Evolution.
SIEA	: Superficial Inferior Epigastric Artery.
SIGAM	: Special Interest Group of Amputee Medicine.
SIGN	: Scottish Intercollegiate Guidelines Network.
SIH	: Spontaneous Intracranial Hypotension.
SIJ	: Sacro-Illiac Joint.
SIJS	: Sacro-Iliac Joint Syndrome.
SIL	: Squamous Intraepithelial Lesion.
SIMV	: Synchronised Intermittent Mandatory Ventilation.
SIP	: Sickness Impact Profile.

Sympathetic Independent Pain.
SIPPV : Synchronized Intermittent Positive Pressure Ventilation.
SIRC : Social Issues Research Centre.
SIRES : Stabilise, Identify Toxin, Reverse effect, Eliminate toxin, Support.
SIRS : Systemic Inflammatory Response Syndrome.

SJDC : Scottish Junior Doctors Committee.
SJO₂. : Oxygen Saturation of Jugular mixed-venous Blood.
SJS : Stevens-Johnson Syndrome.

SL : Scapular Line. (USA).
SL(s.l) : Sublingual.
SLA : Service Level Agreement.
Soluble Liver Antigen.
SLAM : Simultaneous Latram and Mastectomy.
SLAP : Superior Labrum Anterior-to-Posterior.
SLD : Specific Learning Disabilities.
SLE : Systemic Lupus Erythematosus.
SLED : Slow Low-Efficiency Dialysis.
SLEDD : Slow Extended Daily Dialysis.
SLI : Specific Language Impairment.
SLIT : Sublingual Immuno-Therapy.
SLN : Sentinal Lymph Node.
SLOB : Same Lingual Opposte Buccal.(Ref. movements of **Parallax** in Radiology).
SLR : Straight Leg Raise (or Raising)..
SLS : Selected List Scheme.
Social and Life Skills.
SLT : Single Lung Transplant.
Speech and Language Therapy.

SM : Substance Misuse.
Systolic Murmur.
SMA : Spinal Muscular Atrophy (Type 11). (Ref. an inherited peripheral motor neurone disorder).
Superior Mesenteric Artery.
SMAC : Standing Medical Advisory Committee.

SMART	: Salmeterol Multicentre Asthma Research Trial. (Ref in the **USA**). Specific Measurable acceptable Realistic Timebound (Action). (Ref. a Teaching method).
SMAS	: Superficial Musculo-aponeurotic System.
SMBG	: Self-Monitoring of Blood Glucose.
SMC	: Scottish Medicines Consortium.
SMD	: Standardised Mean Difference. (Ref. in Statistics). Submucus Diathermy (to inferior turbinates).
SMEC	: Student Medical Education Committee.
SMIT	: Society for Minimally Invasive Therapy. (USA).
SMO	: Senior Medical Officer.
SMP	: Sympathetically Mediated (or Maintained) Pain.
SMR	: Standardised Mortality Ratio. Sub-Mucus-Resection.
SMS	: Supramaximal Stimulation.
SMTT	: Spinal Manipulative Thrust Technique.
SMV	: Spiral Vein of Modiolus. Synchronised Mandatory Ventilation.
SMWLMs	: Spinal Mobilisation with Limb Movements.
Sn	: Snellen (Test type).
SN	: Saphenous Nerve School Nurse. Student Nurse.
SNAC	: Scaphoid Non-union Advanced Collapse.
SNAGs	: Sustained Natural Apophyseal Glides.
SNAP	: Sensory Nerve Action Potential.
SNB	: Scottish National Board (for Nursing, Midwifery and Health Visiting).
SNHL	: Sensorineural Hearing Loss.
SNMAC	: Standing Nursing and Midwifery Advisory Committee.
SNO	: Senior Nursing Officer.
SNOM	: Selective Non-Operative Management.
SNOMED	: Systematised Nomenclature of Medicine.
SNP	: Sodium Nitroprusside.
SNPs	: Single Nucleotide Polymorphisms
SNRI	: Serotonin and Noradrenaline Re-uptake Inhibitor.

SNRT	: Sinus Node Recovery Time.
SNS	: Somatic Nervous System. (USA).
	Sympathetic Nervous System.
SO₄ ++	: Sulphate.
SOA	: Swelling of Ankles.
SOAP	: Subjective, Objective, Assessment Plan.
SOB	: Short (or Shortness) of Breath.
SOBAR	: Shortness of Breath at Rest.
SOBOE	: Short (or Shortness) of Breath on Exertion.
SOD	: Superoxide Dismutase (Activity).
SOFA	: Sepsis-related Organ Failure Assessment.
	Sequential Organ Failure Assessment.
SOHND	: Supra-Omohyoid Neck Dessection.
SOL	: Space Occupying Lesion.
SOLVD	: Studies of Left Ventricular Dysfunction.
SOM	: Secretory Otitis Media.
	Serous Otitis Media.
SOMI	: Sterno-Occipital-Mandibular Immobiliser.
	Serious Otitis Media Infection.
SON	: Subject`s Own Name.
SOOF	: Sub-Orbicularis Oculi Fat.
SOPs	: Standard Operating Procedures.
	Surgical Outpatients.
SOPD	: Surgical Outpatients Department.
SOS	: Supplementary Ophthalmic Service.
	Symptoms of Stress (Inventory).
SOVA	: Sinus of Valsalva Aneurysm.
Sp	: Spleen.
SP	: Saphenopopliteal.
SP-1	: Pregnancy-specific beta-1 glycoprotein.
SPA	: Scottish Prescribing Authority.
	Sphenopalatine Artery.
	Supporting Professional Activity.
	Suprapubic Aspiration (of Urine).
SPAD	: Single—Pass Albumin Dialysis.

SPADI	: Shoulder Pain and Disability Index.
SPAPCC	: Scottish Partnership Agency for Palliative and Cancer Care.
SPD	: Symphesis Pubis Dysfunction.
SPC (SmPC)	: Summary of Product Characteristics.
SpCO	: Non-Invasive Carboxyhaemoglobin. (Ref. **MASIMO** monitoring).
SPECT	: Single Proton Emission Computed Tomography.
SPEP	: Serum Protein Electrophoresis.
SPET	: Single Proton Emission Tomography.
SPF	: Sun Protection Factor.
SPG	: Sphenopalatine Ganglion.
SpHb	: Non-Invasive total Haemoglobin (by **MASIMO** monitoring).
SPIN	: Scale of Pain Intensity.
SPK	: Simultaneous Pancreas and Kidney.
SpMet.	: Non-Invasive Methaemoglobin-measurement.(Using **MASIMO** monitoring).
SpO2	: Peripheral Oxygen saturation.
SPOA	: Subperiosteal Orbital Abscess.
SpO2C	: Non-Invasive Oxygen Content-measurement.(Using **MASIMO** monitoring).
Spp.	: Species.
SPQ	: Specialist Practitioner Qualification.
SpR	: Specialist Registrar.
SPSS	: Statistical Package for Social Sciences.
Spt	: Spirit. Sputum.
SPT	: Skin Prick Test. (Ref. in Allergy testing).
SPV	: Systolic Pressure Variation.
SQI	: Signal Quality Index.
SQUIRE	: Standard for Quality Improvement Reporting Excellence.
SR	: Sinus Rhythm. Slow Release. Steroid Resistant. Sustained Release.

SRD	: Specific Reading Disability.
	State Registered Dietician; (now called Registered Dietician; **RD**).
SRE	: Sex and Relationship Education.
SROM	: Spontaneous Rupture of the Membranes.
SRIs	: Serotonin Re-uptake Inhibitors.
SRN	: State Registered Nurse.
SRNS	: Steroid Responsive Nephrotic Syndrome.
SRSV	: Small Round-Structured Virus.
SRY	: Sex-Related Y (gene).
Ssc	: Systemic Sclerosis.
SS	: Steroid-Sensitive.
	Systemic Sclerosis.
SSA	: Swallow-Screening Assessment.
SSC	: Somatic Stem Cell.
	Superior Semi-circular Canal.
SSEIs	: Selective Serotonin re-uptake Inhibitors.
SSEP	: Somato-Sensory Evoked Potential.
SSFO	: Safe, Simple and Fast Oxygenation.
SSI	: Social Services Inspectorate.
	Surgical Stimulation Index.
SSLMA	: Soft Seal Laryngeal Mask Airway.
SSM	: Special Study Module.
SSP	: Statutory Sick Pay.
SSPE	: Subacute Sclerosing Pancephalitis.
SSRB	: Seniors Salary Review Body.
SSRC	: Social Science Research Council.
SSRIs	: Selective Serotonin Re-uptake Inhibitors.
SSRO	: Sagittal Split Ramus Osteotomy.
SSS	: Staford Sleepness Scale.
	Staphylococcal Scalded Skin Syndrome.
	"Slipping Slipper Sign" (Ref. in Diabetic Peripheral Neuropathy).
SSSS	: Staphylococcal Scalded Skin Syndrome.
SST	: Stereotactic Subcaudate Tractotomy.
ST	: Sanitary Towel.

Specialist Training (Trainee.)
Speech Therapist.
Stomach.
Surgical Tracheostomy.

STA : Specialist Training Authority.

STAF : Strategies of Treatment of Atrial Fibrillation.

STAI : Spielberger State-Trait Anxiety Inventory. (Ref. baseline data for surgical patients).

STAN : ST-Analysis of the Foetal Electrocardiogram (**ECG**).

STAR : Steming the Tide of Antibiotic Resistance.

STARD : Sequenced Treatment Alternatives to Relieve Depression.

START : Simple Triangle and Rapid Treatment.

STAT : Supra-Threshold Adaptation Test.

Stat. : Statim. (Ref. Latin for; "At once/immediately").

STD : Sexually Transmitted Disease.
Sodium Tetradecyl Sulphate.

STE : S-T Elevation. (Ref. on the **ECG**).
Subperiosteal Tissue Expander.

STEMI : S-T Elevation Myocardial Infarct.

STEPS : System for Thalidomide Education and Prescribing Safety. (USA).

STF : Superficial Temporal Fascia.

STH : Somatotropic Hormone.

STIs : Sexually Transmitted Infections.

STIR : Short tau inversion recovery (sequences.) (Ref. sequences during **MRI).**

STLA : Sub-Teno`s Local Anaesthesia.

STM : Short-Term Memory.

STOP : Surgical Termination of Pregnancy.

STP : Standard Temperature and Pressure.

STPD : Standard Temperature and Pressure Dry.

STS : Serological Test for Syphilis.

STSG : Split-Thickness Skin Graft.

STSS : Streptococcal Toxic Shock Syndrome.

SUA : Serum Uric Acid.

SUDEP : Sudden Unexpected Death in Epilepsy.

SUDI : Sudden Unexpected Death of an Infant.

SUFE	: Slipped Upper Femoral Epiphysis.
SUNCT	: Short-lasting, Unilateral, Neuralgiform headache with Conjuctival Injection, Tearing, rhinorrhoea and forehead sweating (syndrome).
Sup.	: Superior.
Supf.	: Superficial.
SUZI	: Subzonal Insemination.
Sv	: Splenic vein.
SV	: Saphenous Vein.
	Splenic Vessels.
	Spontaneous Ventilation.
	Stroke Volume.
SVC	: Superior Vena Cava.
SVCO	: Superior Vena Caval Obstruction.
SVD	: Simple Vertex Delivery.
	Spontaneous Vertex Delivery.
	Spontaneous Vaginal Delivery.
SVE	: Sterile Vaginal Examination.
SVG	: Saphenous Vein Graft.
SV(I)	: Stroke Volume (Index).
Svt	: Synchronous Ventilation.
SVR	: Systemic Vascular Resistance.
SVRI	: Systemic Vascular Resistance Index.
SVT	: Supraventricular Tachycardia.
SVV	: Stroke Volume Variation.
SWD	: Short-Wave Diathermy.
SWOT	: Strength, Weakness, Opportunities, Threats. (Ref. alcoholism assessment).
SWP	: South West Regional Council.(Ref. Strategic Health Authority and **NHS** Finances).
SWS	: Slow Wave Sleep.
Sxs	: Symptoms.
SXR	: Skull X-Ray.
Sy (Syph)	: Syphilis.

Sy(n)	: Syndrome.
SZS	: Seizures.
T	: Temperature.
	Term.
	Thorax.
	Treatment.
Ts	: Tonsils (or Tonsillectomy).
T3	: Triiodothyronine.
T4	: Tetra-iodo-thyronine (or Thyroxine).
T1–12	: Thoracic Spine Segments/Thoracic Ribs.
T13	: Trisomy 13.
T18	: Trisomy 18.
T21	: Trisomy 21.
TA	: Temporal Arteritis.
	Terminologia Anatomica.
	Tibialis Anterior.
	Transabdominal.
	Tricuspid Atresia.
	Triple Antigen.
TA-4	: Tumour Associated Antigen.
TAA	: Thoracic Aortic Aneurysm.
	Total Ankle Arthroplasty.
TAAA	: Thoraco-Abdominal Aortic Aneurysm.
Ts & As	: Tonsils and Adenoids.
Tab	: Tablet.
TAB	: Typhoid-Paratyphoid A and B (Vaccine).
TAB+Cho.	: Typhoid-Paratyphoid A, B, (Vaccine) + Cholera (Vaccine).
TABC	: Typhoid-Paratyphoid A, B, and C vaccine.
TABT	: Typhoid-Paratyphoid A, and B with Tetanus Toxoid.
TAC	: Time, Amount, Character.
TACE	: Trans-arterial Chemo-Embolisation.
TACS	: Total Anterior Circulation Stroke.
TADS	: Treatment for Adolescents with Depression Study.
TAGs	: Therapeutic Advisory Groups. (USA).
TaGVHD	: Transfusion-Associated Graft versus Host Disease.
TAH	: Total Abdominal Hysterectomy.

TAH+BSO	: Total Abdominal Hysterectomy and Bilateral Salpingo-Oophorectomy.
TAP	: Test for Attentional Performance. (Ref. attention and memory test). Transversus Abdominis Plain (Block).
TAPVD	: Total Anomalous Pulmonary Venous Drainage.
TAR	: Thrombocytopenia-Absent Radius (Syndrome).
TARN	: Trauma Audit and Research Network.
TAS	: Trans-Abdominal Scan.
TASH	: Transcoronary Ablation of Septal Hypertrophy.
TAMBA	: Twins and Multiple Births Association.
TAMPA	: Tampa Scale for Kinesiophobia.
TAT	: Turn Around Time.(Ref. Time between sampling and getting test results). Thrombin-Antithrombin 111 (complexes).
TATc	: Thrombin-Anti-Thrombin Complex.
TB	: Tubercle Bacillus (Tuberculosis).
TBA	: To Book Again. To be advised.
TBAH	: Tetra-n-butyl-Ammonium Hydroxide.
TBC	: Traumatic Bone Cyst.
TBG	: Thyroxine-binding Globulin.
TBI	: Total Body Irradiation. Traumatic Brain Injury.
TBIDA	: Trimethylbromoiminodiacetic Acid.
Tbil.	: Total Bilirubin.
TBK	: Total Body Potassium.
TBL	: Total Blood Loss.
TBLR	: Transconjuctival Blepharoplasty Laser Resurfacing.
TBM	: Tuberculous Meningitis.
TBNA	: Trans-Bronchial Needle Aspiration.
TBPA	: Thyroid Binding Pre-Albumin.
TBSA	: Total Body Surface Area.
TBT	: Transcervical Balloon Tuboplasty.
TBW	: Tatol Body Water. Total Body Weight.

Tc	: Technetium.
TC	: Total Cholesterol.
3TC	: Lamivudine.
TCA	: Target Controlled Anaesthesia.
	To-Come-Again.
	Trichloroacetic Acid.
	Tricyclic Antidepressants.
TCAD	: Tricyclic Anti-Depressant.
TCC	: Transitional Cell Carcinoma.
TCD	: Trans-cranial Doppler. (Ref. in Ultrasonography).
TCDB	: Trauma Coma Data Bank.
TcES	: Trans-cranial Electrical Stimulation.(Ref. monitoring during surgery for **TAAA** and **TTAA**).
TCI	: Target Controlled Infusion.
	To-Come-In.
TCM	: Traditional Chinese Medicine.
TCN	: Take Care Now.(Ref. Locum **GP** Agency for **OOH** service cover).
TcCO$_2$	: Transcutaneous Carbon Dioxide Pressure.
TcO$_2$	: Transcutaneous Oxygen Pressure.
TcPO$_2$.	: Transcutaneous Oxygen Tension.
TCP	: Thrombocytopenia.
TCR	: T-Cell Receptor.
	Trigeminal Cardiac Reflex.
TCRE	: Transcervical Resection of the Endometrium.
TCS	: Terms and Conditions of Service.
	Transforming Community Services.
TCT	: Thrombin Clotting Time.
TD	: Tardive Dyskinesia.
TDD	: Total Digitalising Dose (of Digoxin).
TDE	: Tissue-Doppler Echocardiography.
TDGF	: Thrombin-derived Growth Factor.
TDI	: Transition Dyspnoea Index.
TDM	: Therapeutic Drug Monitoring.
T$_1$DM	: Type 1 Diabetes Mellitus.
T$_2$DM	: Type 2 Diabetes Mellitus.

TDR	: Transmural Dispersion of Repolarisation.(Ref. in Cardiac repolarisation).
tds	: Ter die sumendum. (Ref. Latin for; "three times a day").
TDS	: Three times a day. (Ref. see under **t.d.s**). Testosterone Deficiency Syndrome.
TDT	: Trieger Dot Test. (Ref. a measure of psychomotor function).
TE	: Expiratory Time. Tracheo-oesophageal.
TEA	: Thoracic Epidural Analgesia. Total Elbow Arthroplasty.
TEB	: Thoracic Electrical Bio-impedance.
TED	: Thrombo-embolic Deterrents. Thrombo-embolic Disease.
TEDS	: Thrombo-embolic Deterrent Stockings.
TEE	: Thoracic Expansion Exercises. Total Energy Expenditure. Transesophageal Echocardiography. (USA).
TEER	: Trans-Epitherial Electrical Resistance.
TEG	: Thrombo-Elastography. (Ref. in Platelet mapping).
TEM	: Technical Error of Measurement.
TEMDI	: The European Medical Directory.
TEN	: Toxic Epidermal Necrolysis.
TENS	: Transcutaneous Electrical Nerve Stimulation.(Ref. test for neuro-muscular block and in Pain management).
TEP	: Tracheoesophageal Puncture.
TERIS	: Teratogen Information Service.(Ref. Teratogen Drug effects and risks).
TES	: Therapeutic Error Signal. Trans-Thoracic Endoscopic Sympathectomy.
TESA	: Testicular Epididymal Sperm Aspiration.
TESE	: Testicular Sperm Extraction.
Tet.	: Tetanus. Tetracycline.
Tet/Ser.	: Tetanus Antitoxin.
Tet/Vac.	: Tetanus Toxoid.

TF	: Tissue Factor.
	Transdermal Fentanyl.
	Transferrin.
TFA	: Trifluoroacetic Acid.
TFCC	: Triangular Fibrocartilage Complex.
TFL	: Tail-Flick Latency.
	Transnasal Fiberoptic Laryngoplasty.
TFNs	: Tonically-firing Neurones. (Ref. Dorsal Spinal Neurones).
TFP	: Temporalis Fascia Proper.
TFPI	: Tissue Factor Pathway Inhibitor.
TfR	: Transferrin Receptor.
TFTs	: Thyroid Function Tests.
TG	: Triglycerides.
Tg	: Thyroglobulin.
TGA	: Transient Global Amnesia.
	Transposition of the Great Arteries.
TGC	: Temperature Gradient Correction.
TGDC	: Thyroglossal Duct Cyst.
TGF	: Transforming Growth Factor.
TGT	: Thromboplastic Generation Time.
TGV	: Transposition of the Great Vessels.
THA	: Total Hip Arthroplasty.
THC	: (Delta-9)-Tetrahydro-Cannabinol.(Ref. the content of in Cannabis).
THelpe	: Thymus Lymphocytes.
THET	: Tropical Health and Education Trust.
THIN	: The Health Improvement Network (Database.)
THPA	: Treponema pallidum Haemagglutination Assay.
THR	: Total Hip Replacement (or Arthroplasty).
	Transient Hyperaemic Response. (Ref. in cerebral autoregulation).
ThV	: Thoracic Vertebra.
TI	: Inspiratory Time.
	Tricuspid Incompetence.

TIA	: Transient Ischaemic Attack.
TIBC	: Total Iron-binding Capacity.
TICS	: Telephone Interview for Cognitive Status.
TID	: Type 1 Diabetes. (Ref. Juvenile Diabetes.)
TID (tid; tds)	: Ter in die. (Ref. Latin for; "three times a day").
TIF	: Tracheal Innominate (Artery) Fistula.
TIMI	: Thrombosis in Myocardial Infarction.
TIMPs	: Tissue Inhibitor of Metallo-Proteinases.
TIPS	: Teaching Improvement Programme System.
	Transjugular Intrahepatic Portosystemic Stent.
	Transjugular Intrahepatic Portosystemic Shunting.
TIPSS	: Transjugular Intrahepatic Portasystemic Shunts.
TIsegment	: Thoracic Spinal segment.
TISS	: Thapeutic Intervention Scoring System.
TITs	: Trimming of the Inferior Turbinates.
TIVA	: Total Intravenous Anaesthesia.
TIWR	: Tetanic Stimulus-Induced Withdraw Reflex. (Ref. study of Anaesthetic Drugs effect on the Spinal Cord).
TJP	: Tracheo-Jejunal Puncture.
TKA	: Total Knee Arthroplasty.
TKco	: Transfer co-efficient.
TKI	: Tyrosine Kinase Inhibitor.
TKJR	: Total Knee Joint Replacement.
TKR	: Total Knee Replacement (or Arthroplasty).
TKVO	: To Keep Vein Open.
TLC	:"Tender Loving Care." (Ref. providing analgesia in terminal care).
	Thin-layer Chromatography.
	Total Lung Capacity.
	Total Lymphocyte Count.
TLD	: Thermo-luminescent Dosimeter. (Ref. Lithium Fluoride badges for monitoring and measuring Radiation dose).
TLE	: Temporal Lobe Epilepsy.
TLOSR	: Transient Lower Oesophageal Sphincter Relaxations.
TLP	: Total Laryngopharyngectomy.
TLR	: Toll-Like Receptors.

TLSO	: Thoraco-Lumbar Sacral Orthosis.
TLV	: Two Lung Ventilation.
TM	: Tympanic Membrane.
TMA	: Transcription-Mediated Amplification.
T.major	: Teres major.
TMC	: Total Morphine Consumption.(Ref. in Patient-controlled Morphine Analgesia administration).
TMJ	: Temporo-Mandibular Joint.
TMPDS	: Temporomandibular Pain Dysfunction Syndrome.
TMPG	: Transmural Pressure Gradient.(Ref. to cerebral aneurysm measurement).
TMR	: Transmyocardial Laser Revascularisation. Transmyocardial Revascularisation.
TMRP	: Transmembrane Regulator Protein.
TMS	: Transcranial Magnetic Stimulation.
Tn-1	: Troponin 1.
Tn-1 (cTn-1)	: Cardiac Troponin 1
TN	: Temperature Normal. Trigeminal Neuralgia.
TNF	: Tumour Necrosis Factor.
TNFa	: Tumour Necrosis Factor alpha.
TNM (T/N/M)	: Tumour, Node, Metastasis.(Ref. classification and staging of Tumours).
TNR	: True Negative Rate.
TNT	: Treatment to New Targets.
TnT (cTnT)	: Cardiac Troponin T.
TOA	: Tubo-Ovarian Abscess.
TOBEC	: Total Body Electrical Conductivity.
TOC	: Transvaginal Oviductal Cannulation.
TOE	: Transoesophageal Echocardiogram (or Echocardiography).
ToF	: Train of Four. (Ref. test for neuro-muscular block recovery).
TOF	: Tetralogy of Fallot. Tracheo-oesophageal Fistula.

Train of Four. (Ref. Test for level of muscle relaxation in Anaesthesia).

TOFR : Train of Four Ratio. (Ref. used in Anaesthesia).

TOMBOLA : Trial of Management of Borderline and Low Grade Abnormal Smears).

TOP : Termination of Pregnancy.
Treatment Outcome Profile.

TOR : Termination of Resuscitation.

TORCH : Toxoplasmosis,Others,Rubella, Cytomegalovirus, Herpes simplex and Hepatitis B.

TORP : Total Ossicular Reconstruction Prothesis.

TOS : Thoracic Outlet Syndrome.

TP : Total Protein.

TPA(Tpa) : Tissue-type Plasminogen Activator.

TP(TwPmo.) : Twitch mouth Pressure.

TPE : Total Protein Excretion (Urinary).

TPHA : Treponema Pallidum Haemagglutination Assay.

TPI : Treponema Pallidum Immobilisation (Test).

TPMT : Thiopurine Methyl Transferase.

TPN : Total Parenteral Nutrition.

TPO : Thyroid Peroxidase.

TPOAb : Thyroid Peroxidase Antibodies.

TPP : Thiamine Pyrophosphate

TPR (T/P/R) : Temperature, Pulse, Respiration.
Total Peripheral Resistance.
True Positive Rate.

TPS : Thiopenton Sodium. (Ref. a Barbiturate drug used in Anaesthesia).

TPSE : Tricuspid Annular Plane Systolic Excursion.

TPT : Thermal Softened Preformed Tube. (Ref. type of Anaesthetic **ETTube**).

TPV : Triple Polio Vaccine.

TR : Tricuspid (Valve) Regurgitation.

TRAB : Thyrotrophin Receptor Antibodies.

TRALI : Transfusion-Related Acute Lung Injury.

TRAM : Transverse Rectus Abdominis Myocutaneous (flap).

TRAP	: Twin Reversed Arterial Perfusion.
TRAIU	: Thyroid Radioactive Iodine Uptake.
TRCC	: Transfusion Requirements in Critical Care.
TRD	: Tinnitis-Relief Device.
TRE	: Temporary Registration in an Emergency. (Ref. by the **GMC**).
TREDs	: Trinucleotide Repeat Expansion Diseases.
TRH	: Thyrotrophin-releasing Hormone (or Thyroid-Releasing Hormon.
TRIM	: Transfusion Related Immuno-Modulation.(Ref. to altered characteristics of T-lymphocytes by Blood Transfusion.)
TRISS	: Trauma Injury Severity Score.
TRCL	: Total Red Blood Cell Loss.
TRP	: Tubular Reabsorption of Phosphate.
TRU	: Trauma Resuscitation Unit.
TRUS	: Trans-Rectal Ultrasound Scan. Transrectal Ultraonography.
TS	: Tanner Stages (1–5 in Puberty). Tourette's (or Gilles de la) Syndrome. (Ref. psychiatric disorders like **ADHD** and **OCD**). Tricuspid (Valve) Stenosis.
TSA	: Total Shoulder Arthroplasty.
TSAA	: Tri-Service Anaesthetic Apparatus.
TSC	: Technical Steering Committee. Tuberous Sclerosis Complex.
TSCN	: Registered Sick Children's Nurse.
TSE	: Testicular Self-Examination. Transmissible Spongiform Encephalopathies.
TSF	: Triceps Skin Fold (Thickness).
TSFS	: Trans-Septal-Frontal Sinusotomy.
TSGs	: Tumour Suppressor Genes.
TSH	: Thyroid Stimulating Hormone.
TSIg	: Thyroid Stimulating Immunoglobulin.
TSS	: Total Surgical Stress. Toxic Shock Syndrome.
TSSD	: Theatre Sterile Supplies Department.
TSST-1	: Toxic Shock Syndrome Toxin type 1.
TST	: Tuberculin Skin Test.

Triceps Skinfold Thickness. (see **TSF**).

T-tube : Long-term Grommet.
TT : Tetanus Toxoid.
Thrombin Time. (see Thrombin Clotting Time **TCT**).
Tracheal Tube.
Tuberculin Tested.
TTA : Torn Tendon Archilles.
TTAs :"To take aways." (Ref. discharge drugs).
TTAA : Trans-Thoracic Aortic Aneurysm.
TTB : Tetanus Toxoid Booster.
TTC : Triphenyl-Tetrazolium Chloride.(Ref. Laboratory staining solution).
TTD : Tissue Tracking Displacement. (Ref. in Propofol Anaesthesia).
TTDI : Thoretical Toxic Dose Index.
TTE : Trans-Thoracic Echocardiogram (or Cardiography)..
TTFM : Transit Time Flow Meter.(Ref. used to assess blood flow in surgical Free Flaps).
TTH : To Take Home.
TTJV : Trans-Tracheal Jet Ventilation.
TTKG : Transtubular Potassium Gradient.
TTN : Transient Tachypnoea of the Newborn.
TTOs :"To take outs." (Ref. discharge drugs.)
TTP : Tender to Percussion.
Thrombotic Thrombocytopenic Purpura.
TTS : Temporary Threshold Shift.
Tissue Tracking Score.(Ref. Propofol Anaesthesia and **LVF**).
TTTS : Twin-Twin Transfusion Syndrome.
TTX : Tetrodotoxin. (Ref. a Sodium channel blocker.)

TUE : Therapeutic Use Exemption.
TUPASS : Tuebingen Centre for Patient Safety and Stimulation.
TUR : Trans-Urethral Resection.
TURBT : Transurethral Resection of Bladder Tumour.
TURP : Trans-Uretheral Resection of the Prostate.

TV	: Tidal Volume. (see **Vt**).
	Transvaginal.
	Transverse (position of Foetus).
	Trichomonas Vaginalis.
	Tricuspid Valve.
TVM	: Trans-Vaginal Monitoring. (Ref. in Obstetrics).
TVR	: Tonic Vibrating Reflex.
TVS	: Transvaginal (Pelvic) Ultrasound.
TVT	: Trans-Vaginal Tape.
	Tension-free Vaginal Tape.
TWA	: Time-Weighted Average.
TWOC	: Trial Without Catheter.
TwPdi.	: Twitch Trans-diaphragmatic Pressure.
TwPet.	: Twitch Tracheal Tube Pressure.
TwPoes.	: Twitch Oesophageal Pressure.
Tx	: Thromboxane.
	Treatment.
TXA	: Tranexamic Acid.
TYM	: Test Your Memory.
TZ	: Transitional (or Transformation) Zone.
TZD	: Thiazolidinediones (Drugs).
U	: Umbilical.
	Unit.
	Urea.
	Urethra.
U 11	: Urotensin 11. (Ref. an endogenous vasoconstrictor).
UA	: Umbilical Artery.
	Unstable Angina.
	Urinalysis.
UAC	: Umbilical Arterial Catheter.
UB	: Urinary Bladder.

UC	: Ulcerative Colitis.
UCAS	: University and Colleges Administration Service.
UCC	: Uniform Commercial Code. (USA).
UCC	: Urgent Care Cambridge.(Ref. local **GPs** Consortium for **OOH** cover).
UCE	: Upper-Completely Edentulous.
U,C+E	: Urea, Creatinine and Electrolytes.
UCL	: Ulna Collateral Ligament.
UCR	: Usual and Customary Rate. (USA).
UDCA	: Ursodeoxycholic Acid. (Ref. in Cardiac Failure).
UDGT	: Uridine-Diphospho-Glucuronyl-Transferase.(Ref. also known as **UGT**).
UDP	: Uridine Diphosphoglucuronate.
UDVs	: Uni-Directional Valves. (Ref. in Anaesthetic Breathing Circle System).

U & Es (U+Es): Urea and Electrolytes.	
uE3.	: Unconjugated Oestriol.
UEMS	: Union of European Medical Specialists.
UES	: Upper Oesophageal Sphincter.
UFH	: Un-Fractionated Heparin.
UG	: Urogenital.
UGH	: Uveitis, Glaucoma, Hyphaemia (Syndrome).
UGS	: Urogenital System.
UGT	: Urogenital Tract.
UHT	: Ultra-Heat Treatment.
UICP	: Universal Infection Control Precautions.
UIP	: Usual Interstitial Pneumonia.
UKCAT	: United Kingdom Clinical Aptitude Test.
UKCC	: United Kingdom Central Council (for Nursing, Midwifery and Health Visiting).
UKFPO	: United Kingdom Foundation Programme Office.
UKMI	: United Kingdom Medicines Information (Service).

UKMIPG	: United Kingdom Medicines Information Pharmacists Group.
UKNP	: United Kingdom National Poisons.
UKPDS	: United Kingdom Prospective Diabetes Study.
UL	: Upper Limb.
ULN	: Upper Limit of Normal.
ULNT	: Upper Limb Neurodynamic Test.
ULS	: Upper Labial Segment.
ULTRA	: Unrelated Liver Transplant Regulatory Authority.
ULTT	: Upper Limb Tension Test.
UM	: Ultra-rapid Metaboliser..
UMN	: Upper Motor Neurone.
UMNL	: Upper Motor Neurone Lesions.
UNC	: Urine Net Charge.
UNHS	: Universal Neonatal Hearing Screening.
UO	: Urine Output.
UPDRS	: Unified Parkinson`s Disease Rating Scale.
UPEP	: Urine Protein Electrophoresis.
UPSI	: Un-Protected Sexual Intercourse.
UPT	: Urine Pregnancy Test.
UP: UCr	: Urinary Protein to Urinary Creatinine (ratio).
URA	: Upper Removable Appliance
URIs	: Upper Respiratory Tract Infections.
UR-NAP	: Urea-Resistant Neutrophil Alkaline Phosphatase.
UROL	: Urology.
URT	: Upper Respiratory Tract.
URTI	: Upper Respiratory Tract Infection.
US (U/S)	: Ultrasound.
USFDA	: United States Food and Drug Administration.
USNIDA	: United States National Institute on Drug Abuse.
USP	: United States Pharmacopoeia.

USS	: Ultrasound Scan(ning).
UST	: Upper Single Tooth.
Ut	: Uterus
UT	: Un-Trained.
	Urinary Tract.
UTI	: Urinary Tract Infection.
UUTI	: Uncomplicated Urinary Tract Infection.
UV	: Ultraviolet.
UVA	: Ultraviolet A.
UVB	: Ultra-Violet B. (Ref. in Phototherapy).
UVC	: Umbilical Vein Catheter.
UVL	: Ultraviolet Light.
UVmax	: (Maximum) Umbilical Vein Velocity.
UVprolapse	: Utero-Vaginal Prolapse.
UVPPP	: Uvulopalatopharyngoplasty.
UVR	: Ultraviolet Radiation.
UWS	: University of Wales Swansea.
UZ	: Upper Zone.
V	: Vagina.
	Variable.
	Vein.
	Visit.
Va (VA)	: (Alveolar) Ventilation.
VA	: Visual Acuity.
	Visual Analogue.
Vac.	: Vaccination.
VAC	: Vacuum-Assisted Closure. (Ref. Wound closure after debridement).
VACTERL	: Vertebral, Anal, Cardiac, Tracheal, Oesophageal, Renal and Limb.
VaD	: Vascular Dementia.
VAD	: Ventricular-Assisted Devices.

VADS	: Visual Aural Span (Test).
VAE	: Venous Air Embolism.
VA-ECMO	: Veno-Arterial Extracorporeal Membrane Oxygenation.
Vag.	: Vaginitis.
VAIN	: Vaginal Intraepithelial Neoplasia.
VAP	: Ventilator Associated Pneumonia.
VAPS	: Visual Analogue Pain Scores.
VARS	: Visual Aura Rating Scale.
VAS	: Vegetative State.
	Visual Analogue Scale.
VATER	: Vertebral, Anal, Tracheal, Oesophageal and Renal.
VATS	: Video-Assisted Thoracoscopic Surgery.
VB	: Vertebral Body.
VBAC	: Vaginal Birth After Caesarean Section (Delivery).
VBG	: Vasculised Bone Graft.
VBI	: Vertebrobasilar Insufficiency.
VC	: Vertebral Canal.
	Vital Capacity.
VCAM-1	: Vascular Cell Adhesion Molecule-1.
VCD	: Vocal Cords-Carina Distance.
VCFS	: Velo-Cardio-Facial Syndrome.
VCR	: Villus to Crypt Ratio.
VCUG	: Voiding Cystourethrogram.
Vd	: Volume of distribution.
VD	: Venereal Disease.
VDA	: Vascular Disruptive Agents. (Ref. e.g Combretastatin).
VDanat.	: Anatomical Dead Space.
VDalv.	: Alveolar Dead Space.
VDBB	: Vertical Diagonal Bands of Broca. (Ref. a Brain structure).
VDDR	: Vitamin D-Dependent Rickets.
VDGF	: Vascular-Derived Growth Factor..
VDI	: Vasculitis Damage Index.
VDphys.	: Physiological Dead Space.
VDRL	: Venereal Diseases Research (Reference) Laboratories.

VDRR	: Vitamin D Resistant Rickets.
VDRT	: Venereal Disease Reference Test.
VE	: Vaginal Examination.
	Ventricular Extrasystoles (or Ectopics).
	Vericose Eczema.
VECTOR	: Versatile Endoscopic Capsule for **GIT** Tumour recognition and therapy.
VEGF	: Vascular Endothelial Growth Factor. (see **VDGF**).
VEPs	: Visual Evoked Potentials.
VEs	: Ventricular Extra-systoles.
VF	: Ventricular Fibrillation.
VGE	: Venous Gas Embolism.
VH	: Vaginal Hysterectomy.
VHL	: Von Hippel-Lindau (gene) Disease. (Ref. protein regulating the function of hypoxia-induced Factor: **HIF**).
VI	: Virgo Intacta.
	Visually Impaired.
VIB	: Vertical Infraclavicular Block.
VILI	: Ventilator-Induced Lung Injury.
VIMA	: Volatile Induction and Maintenance of (General) Anaesthesia.
VIN	: Vulval Intraepithelial Neoplasia.
VIP	: Vaso-active Intestinal Polypeptide.
	Ventilation, Infusion, and Pump.
VISA	: Vancomycin-Insensitive Staphylococcus aureus.
vit	: Vitamin.
VLBW	: Very Low Birth Weight.
VLCD	: Very Low Calorie Diet.
VLDL	: Very Low Density Lipoproteins.
VLPs	: Virus-like Particles.
VLS	: Volume Loading Steps. (Ref. in Haemodynamic Measurements).

VMA	: Vanillymandelic Acid.
VMI	: Very Much Improved.
VMO	: Vastus Medialis Obliquus (muscle).
VNE	: Video Naso-Endoscopy.
vol	: Volume.
VOMIT	: Victim of Medical Investigative Technology.(Ref. e.g in **CT** scanning).
VO	: Verbal Order.
VO₂	: Oxygen Uptake.
VOR	: Vestibulo-Ocular Reflux.
VORP	: Vibrating Ossicular Prothesis.
VOT	: Vascular Occlusion Test.

VP	: Venous Pressure.
VPshunt.	: Ventriculo-Peritoneal Shunt.
VPAP	: Variable Positive Airway Pressure.
VPB	: Ventricular Premature Beat.

V/Q	: Ventilation-Perfusion Configuration Ratio (in Lung Scanning).

VR	: Venous Return.
VRE	: Vancomycin-Resistant Enterococci.
VRI	: Vanilloid Receptor Inhibitor.
VRS	: Verbal Rating Scale.

VSD	: Ventricular Septal Defect.
VSS-GBI	: Vascular Surgical Society of Great Britain and Ireland. (GB & Ire).

Vt	: (Tidal) Volume.
VT	: Venous Thrombosis.
	Ventricular Tachycardia.
VTE	: Venous Thrombo-Embolism.
	Venous Thrombolytic Embolism.
VTEC	: Verocytotoxigenic Escherichia.Coli.

VTN	: Vocational Training Number.
VTRC	: Volume of Transfused Red Blood Cells.
VTV	: Volume Targeted Ventilation.

VU	: Vericose Ulcer.
VUJ	: Vesico-Ureteric Junction.
VUR	: Vesico-Ureteric Reflux.

VVs	: Vericose Veins.
VVBP	: Veno-Venous Bypass.
V-VF	: Vesico-Vaginal Fistula.
VVt	: Ventilator Breaths per minute.
vWD	: von Willebrand`s Disease.
vWF	: von Willebrand Factor. (Ref. its effect on coagulation).
VWF	: Vibration White Finger.

Vx	: Vertex.

VZIG(VZIgG)	: Varicella Zoster Immunoglobulin G.
VZV	: Varicella Zoster Virus.

W	: Watt.
	Weekly (Dose).
WADA	: World Anti-Doping Agency.
WAGR	: Wilms, Aniridia, Gonadal dysplasia, Retarded (Complex).
WAIS	: Wechester Adult Intelligence Scale.
WAMBA	: Wise Areolar Mastopexy Breast Augmentation.
WAME	: World Association of Medical Editors.
WAS	: Ward Atmosphere Scale.
WB	: Weight-bearing.
WBC	: White Blood Cells.
WBT	: Wet Bulb Temperature.(Ref. measuring environment temperature load).

WC	: Whooping Cough.
WCC	: White Cell Count.
WCE	: Wireless Capsule Endoscopy.

WCH	: Wales Centre for Health.
WCRF	: World Cancer Research Fund.
WCSC	: Whittington Consultants Support Committee.
WE	: Wernike`s Encephalopathy.
WEP	: Wideband External Pulse.
WFSA	: World Federation of Societies of Anesthesiologists.
WG	: Wegener`s Granulomatosis.
WHI	: Women`s Health Initiative.
WHO	: World Health Organisation.
WHOQOL	: World Health Organisation Quality of Life (Assessment).
WHS	: Women`s Health Study.
WIsH	: Welsh Innovations in Healthcare.
WIPO	: World Intellectual Property Organisation.
Wipp	: Working in partnership Programme (for **HCNs** and **QNs**).
wk**/s**	: Week/s.
WLE	: Wide Local Excision.
WM	: Waldenstrom`s Macroglobulinaemia.
WMA	: World Medical Association.
WMD	: Weighted Mean Difference. (Ref. in Statistical analysis.)
WML	: White Matter Lesions.(Ref. type of Brain lesions in White Matter).
WNB	: Welsh National Board (for Nursing, Midwifery and Health Visiting).
WNCCC	: Women`s National Cancer Control Campaign.
WNL	: Within Normal Limits.
WOB	: Work of Breathing.
WONCA	: World Organisation of National Colleges and Academic Association.

WPW	: Wolff-Parkinson-White Syndrome.
WPWS	: Wolff-Parkinson-White Syndrome.
W/R	: Ward Round.
WR	: Wassermann Reaction.
WRAML	: Wide Range Assessment of Memory and Learning.
WRVS	: Women`s Royal Voluntary Service.
WRWMA	: Worsening Resting Wall Motion Abnormalities.(Ref. diagnosed using Echocardiography).
WS	: Waardenburg`s Syndrome.
WSACS	: World Society of Abdominal Compartment Syndrome.
Wt	: Weight.
WT	: Warthin Tumour. (Ref. benign tumour of the Parotid Gland).
WTD	: Working Time Directive.
XD	: X-linked Dominant.
XDPs	: Cross-linked Fibrin Degradation Products.
XDR	: Extensively Drug Resistant.
Xe	: Xenon.
XEA (XeA)	: Xenon Anaesthesia.
XL	: X-linked (inheritance).
XLH	: X-linked Hypophosphataemic (Rickets.)
X-match	: Cross-match (Blood).
XML	: Extensible Mark-up Language. (Ref. in Anaesthetic Records).
XMRV	: Xenotropic Murine (Leukaemia Virus-related) Virus.
XP	: Xeroderma Pigmentosa. Xiphoid Process.
XR	: (Extensively) Resistant.

	X-linked Recesive. X-ray.
X-RXN	: Cross Reaction.
YAG	: Yttrium-aluminium-garnet (Laser).
YHL	: Years of Healthy Life.
YLL	: Years of Life Lost.
YO	: Year Old.
yr/s	: Year/s.
Z	: Diagnosis.
ZA	: Zondek-Aschheim.
ZDV	: Zidovudine.
Z-E	: Zollinger-Ellison (Syndrome.)
ZFP	: Zero Flow Pressure. (Ref. Cerebral blood flow pressure measurement).
ZIFT	: Zygote Intrafallopian Tube Transfer.
ZIG	: Zoster-Immunoglobulin.
ZMC	: Zygomatico-Maxillary Complex.
ZN	: Ziel-Neelsen (Stain). Ziehl-Neelson (Syndrome).
Zn	: Zinc
ZO	: Zinc Oxide.
ZOE	: Zinc Oxide Eugenol.